A Roller Coaster Ride
With
Brain Injury

(For Loved Ones)

by

Sylvia Behnish

Order this book online at www.trafford.com/08-0107
or email orders@trafford.com

Most Trafford titles are also available at major online book retailers.

© Copyright 2008 Sylvia Behnish.
Edited by Maggie Taylor
Cover Design/Artwork by Kerry Farrell
All rights reserved. No part of this publication may be reproduced, stored in a retrieval system, or transmitted, in any form or by any means, electronic, mechanical, photocopying, recording, or otherwise, without the written prior permission of the author.

Note for Librarians: A cataloguing record for this book is available from Library and Archives Canada at www.collectionscanada.ca/amicus/index-e.html

Printed in Victoria, BC, Canada.

ISBN: 978-1-4251-6964-0

We at Trafford believe that it is the responsibility of us all, as both individuals and corporations, to make choices that are environmentally and socially sound. You, in turn, are supporting this responsible conduct each time you purchase a Trafford book, or make use of our publishing services. To find out how you are helping, please visit www.trafford.com/responsiblepublishing.html

Our mission is to efficiently provide the world's finest, most comprehensive book publishing service, enabling every author to experience success. To find out how to publish your book, your way, and have it available worldwide, visit us online at www.trafford.com/10510

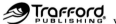 www.trafford.com

North America & international
toll-free: 1 888 232 4444 (USA & Canada)
phone: 250 383 6864 ♦ fax: 250 383 6804 ♦ email: info@trafford.com

The United Kingdom & Europe
phone: +44 (0)1865 722 113 ♦ local rate: 0845 230 9601
facsimile: +44 (0)1865 722 868 ♦ email: info.uk@trafford.com

10 9 8 7 6 5 4 3

Author Biography

Writing has always been a large part of Sylvia's life. She has written two adult fiction novels and a middle grade school fantasy novel. In recent years, she has had many articles published in magazines and newspapers in both Canada and the United States.

A Roller Coaster Ride with Brain Injury (For Loved Ones) is Sylvia's first non-fiction novel. It is written from personal experience and is based on her partner's very serious motorcycle accident and subsequent brain injury.

Sylvia leads a very busy lifestyle. She is actively involved with five grown children and six grandchildren with a seventh due shortly. She also has many interests including photography, gardening, reading and time spent enjoying the wonders of nature.

A special thank you to family and friends for their love and support. We are fortunate to be blessed with an abundance of both.

TABLE OF CONTENTS

Introduction	Page	1
Preface	Page	5
Our First Day In Hell	Page	11
Life Has Changed	Page	18
Changes to Rejoice In	Page	22
Panic Sets In	Page	30
In The Land of the Confused	Page	38
Doing Things His Way	Page	63
Other Changes to Rehabilitation	Page	82
Anger and Frustration	Page	94
Looking After Myself	Page	99
The End of the First Phase	Page	126
Not Taking It Personally	Page	134
Two Steps Forward One Step Back	Page	144
Life Goes On	Page	152
Bumps In The Road	Page	179
Adaptations and Adjustments	Page	188
Epilogue	Page	191
Questions	Page	196
Exercises	Page	202

Introduction

'*A Roller Coaster Ride With Brain Injury (For Loved Ones)*' is a result of Larry, my partner's serious motorcycle accident in August of 2006. When I realized how difficult it was to get information on brain injuries or on how family members can help their brain-injured loved ones, I knew there was a need for something to be written. There seemed to be very little that was readily available for those close to the injured person in learning how to deal with the monumental changes in both the injured person's life and those of his family and friends.

When we are faced with a tragedy such as this, it is difficult to know where to go for answers. Unable to find what I felt I needed, I eventually located the hospital library. I spoke with the librarian and although he said the library was for the use of the hospital staff, he kindly offered to e-mail me several web sites containing information on brain injuries. These were invaluable and were initially my main sources for obtaining information. The web sites are listed at the end of this section.

While Larry was in Royal Columbian Hospital, I found it was also sometimes difficult to get any extensive information from the doctors or the nurses. This was partly because at the beginning very little seemed to be known about the severity of his injury or what the results of the injury would be. I also quickly discovered that what information I was given appeared to be designed to not build up any hopes on my part. Further, I became aware that the more questions I asked, the more variety of answers I received with each person appearing to have a different opinion on both his injury as well as his recovery prognosis.

By writing this book about our situation, I hope to help others in a similar situation realize they are not alone. There will be progress and although it appears to be slow – brain injury progress is often two steps forward and one step back, it will happen. Often the steps are small and changes are sometimes only noticed after a big change has taken place. Moderate brain injury recovery is somewhat like lying awake in the middle of the night feeling like morning will never come – it always does and so also shall there be progress with a moderate brain injury. (In this book I am not dealing with those suffering from severe brain injuries).

There were other reasons why I decided to write a book about Larry's experience. One of these was to assist family members to hopefully be able to understand and know what is involved in being a caregiver. This is difficult since no two head injuries are alike so no two cases will be the same. One of the reasons for this is dependent upon where the head injury occurred (i.e.: is it a frontal lobe injury or....?). Also the personality of the injured person appears to make somewhat of a difference. As a result no two caregivers will experience the exact same problems. There does, however, appear to be some basic similarities.

Another important factor to remember when dealing with a family member who has suffered a brain injury is, that although what has happened is a tragedy for the injured person, it is also a tragedy for his loved ones. As one health care professional told me, 'You must set boundaries for yourself. You are important also'. Often victims of brain injury will be angry and sometimes verbally abusive but as family members and caregivers, we must insist that we be treated with respect also.

Guilt is a big issue. As a family member, it is important that we not allow ourselves to feel guilty when we want time for ourselves, or when we feel angry or upset. We have a right to our feelings. Do not let these feelings of guilt cause you to neglect yourself and your own health.

I found that ICBC (the Insurance Corporation of British Columbia) proved to be an extremely helpful advocate in delivering resources and in directing me to where I might find further assistance. Social Workers in both Royal Columbian Hospital and Queen's Park Care Centre also directed me to places where I might receive help and information.

Being a family member/caregiver requires asking questions because no one will come to you with the answers. I found if I had a concern, I needed to express it. This is very important and necessary if you want to do the best you can in helping your family member become well again. I found most of the medical practitioners were approachable and very willing to listen to my concerns and to help me find a solution – if I asked the questions. It wasn't important however, to just ask the questions, I also had to ask the right questions. It is important also to: 'take control of the situation', 'be proactive' and 'be your own advocate for your family member's brain injury'. I might add, although didn't do myself: contact a Brain Injury Association and speak with others who are going through similar difficult situations. This is particularly important if there is no support from family and friends. I was very fortunate to have both of these support systems in a large measure.

The following are helpful web sites:

For background information:

www.state.sc.us/ddsn/pubs/head/equip.htm
www.neuroskills.com/tbi/bfrontal.shtml
www.waiting.com/frontallobe.html

www.home.iprimus.com.au/rboon/BrainInjury.htm
www.specialtree.com/emotion.behavior.php

For treatment to discuss with your doctor and the rest of the treatment team:

www.health.qld.gov.au/abios/tbi/treat.asp
www.findarticles.com

Preface

When we first met, Larry, a widower of two and a half years with three grown children and one grandchild, wasn't interested in getting into a committed relationship. He spent the first couple of years reliving his 'fun-loving', 'care-free' bachelor days, spending evenings at pubs with friends and weekends cruising the highways on his motorcycle His family, while relatively close, had quite different family dynamics from my own. Special occasions were not particularly celebrated or cared about including Christmas. They may or may not have had a roast beef dinner but a pizza would do just as well. And not a lot of time was spent together socializing as my family did.

I had been divorced for a number of years with no particular interest in a relationship either and for much of that time not even in dating. I had a very busy life with five children and later with grandchildren and many friends and social activities. My family had always been involved with family celebrations and with some of us vacationing and getting together for 'games'. We were and are a family of talkers, much of it engaged in philosophizing and analyzing. I was quite content and happy with my lifestyle and didn't feel there was room in my life for a full-time 'boyfriend'.

Then friends of mine of many years said they knew a man whose wife had died some time ago. They had known him for about twenty-five years – would I be interested in meeting him? I thought there would be no harm in having a male friend for social occasions so, after some thought, I agreed. Getting together with our mutual friends, we discovered almost immediately that we 'clicked'.

Not being a person to rush into anything too quickly, I pondered my serious concern for the fact that he was a smoker. I very nearly decided not to date him because of it. However, we had fun when together and since he came so 'well recommended' by our friends, I continued our friendship on a 'let's see' basis.

Our relationship slowly developed into the close relationship we both later felt fortunate to have. Although we were no 'Spring Chickens', according to our children, we were as excited and happy with our relationship as any two twenty year olds might be.

Initially, we spent many long hours talking and were both amazed that we could spend so much time together enjoying each other's company and conversation without the expectation of anything else at the end of a great evening.

I discovered that Larry was always willing to try a new adventure. In early December, a few months after we met, I asked him if he would like to bring his grandson along to see Christmas lights with me and my grandchildren. He surprisingly agreed, although I don't think looking at Christmas lights was at the top of this 'not long ago' care-free bachelor's list of things to do on a Friday night.

A Roller Coaster Ride With Brain Injury (For Loved Ones)

On another occasion during that month I asked him if he would like to attend my annual cookie exchange. I asked as a lark since it was an all-lady event and didn't expect him to agree. But Larry showed up bringing boxes of chocolate in the correct amount of the cookies required. The annual cookie exchange has since become a 'couple' event.

Each Christmas Eve my family plan a special German traditional dinner with the whole family. I invited him to join us for this special event. He thought a moment and then agreed. Surrounded by about twenty-five people who are demonstrative, talkative and outgoing, I considered him to be quite brave since he had previously met very few of them.

During the first few months, we discovered that we both loved nature and the outdoors and often went on walks and picnics together even when we were into the cold weather months. Our first picnic was on a damp day between Christmas and New Years Day when, although we nearly froze, we laughingly enjoyed our adventure.

We also discovered that both of us were 'artsy', in our own way. Larry is somewhat artistic with his sign making and painting skills and I write, do photography, crafts, paint and enjoy decorating. We worked well together on most projects, particularly on decorating projects; I had the ideas and Larry had many of the skills. Also neither one of us enjoyed watching T.V., preferring instead to be doing things. We both loved to socialize and always had a busy social calendar. The fact that he enjoyed socializing as much as I did further added to the 'glue' of our relationship. I was, and still am, very much an event planner.

It wasn't long before we found that in spite of the many differences in our backgrounds, there was a sameness that made the two halves of our personalities fit together very well into a whole. Larry eventually asked me to move in with him. I hesitated, deciding not to for the same reason I almost decided not to date him in the beginning – because he was a smoker. I said I couldn't live with a smoker. He said he would quit. As a result, he quit and I agreed to move in with him after he had successfully been off cigarettes for four months. It was a big decision on my part.

In the years we had been together, the families blended to some degree. Larry's daughter is around the same age as my daughter and oldest son.

We got along well, rarely disagreeing and when occasionally we did, it was discussed easily and the problem was quickly resolved. Anger in our relationship was never a problem. Our relationship never felt like work; no doubt because we both tended to be easy going with a good sense of humor.

Because our time was flexible, we were able to enjoy long weekends exploring various areas of our beautiful province. On one such trip we visited Gold River. Checking out the town and exploring along the way to take pictures, we suddenly realized how late it was getting and the need to find a camping spot before dark. After searching, we finally found a little used camp site; nearly missing its faded sign among the overgrown trees. Choosing a site on the river side that had less moss covering the picnic table than the rest, we decided to call it 'home' for the night.

Inside the truck where we slept, I pressed various buttons to roll up the windows to keep those pesky mosquitoes out and then slammed the doors shut. After building a camp fire, we went back to the van for the stove and cooler. The doors were all locked!

It was almost dark and we were 45 minutes from civilization and any help. If we couldn't get inside the van to sleep, we'd have been sleeping on the ground but there was no yelling or criticism from Larry. The problem was eventually resolved with the assistance of the only other campers in this backwoods campground who happened to have a whole assortment of keys; one being a Volkswagen key that, with luck, fit our Chevrolet SUV.

The nice thing about the whole experience was that it could have been the beginning of a very unpleasant trip but because we could both see the humor in the situation, a potentially explosive situation turned into a funny story that we've been able to tell friends and family.

We always said we didn't think we'd have a problem that we couldn't talk about and resolve. Life was great!

A Roller Coaster Ride With Brain Injury (For Loved Ones)

Until Larry's accident, this was the case. That is why when it happened I was shocked that I hadn't known the instant it had. I always felt that if something happened to anyone close to me, I would know.

CHAPTER ONE

Our First Day in Hell

August 22

      I didn't know until I received that life-altering phone call. It was the phone call no one ever wants to receive. I had waved goodbye to Larry from the doorway when he left on his motorcycle at 9:30 a.m. on August 22, 2006. I then went into the backyard to paint a lattice we were going to put around the hot tub to give us more privacy from the neighbors. At 10:30 the friend he was supposed to be meeting at 10:00 a.m. phoned to say Larry had not arrived. A faint wave of apprehension washed over me but there was still no major premonition. Although admittedly, he was never late for anything, I pushed the thread of uneasiness away. *Maybe this was one of the rare times he was late. Maybe he had to stop somewhere first and got held up. Maybe traffic was bad. Maybe there was construction.* There were many reasons why someone could be late; I knew them all. I tried to concentrate on my painting.

      At 11:00 a.m. when his friend telephoned again, I could not ignore the uneasiness. Putting the brush down I tried to think of what to do. *Should I drive the route I thought he might have taken? Maybe his motorcycle had broken down. Maybe he had run out of gas.* I didn't try his cell because I knew he couldn't hear the ring above the noise of the motorcycle. I was still pondering the problem when the phone call came at 11:15 a.m.

"Hello, is this Sylvia? My name is Karen. I'm the social worker at the Emergency at Royal Columbian Hospital." As soon as I heard 'Royal Columbian Hospital', I knew immediately that the call had to be very serious because anyone injured in Surrey would normally go to Surrey Memorial Hospital.

I broke down, barely able to speak. She said, "He's alive but it's very serious. Do you have someone who can drive you?"

"I think so." I was barely able to think coherently.

I called my daughter but she said that my grandson had just broken his leg and they had just returned from the hospital. "Oh Mom, I can't move him. He's in so much pain."

Unable to remember how to get to Royal Columbian Hospital, I asked her for directions. My brain had literally turned to mush and any previous knowledge of how to get there had evaporated.

"I'll phone and let everyone know what's happened," she promised.

Unable to stop the floodgate of tears, I cried the whole way to the hospital, praying that Larry would be alive. Finally, after what seemed to be hours later I arrived at the parking lot but was

A Roller Coaster Ride With Brain Injury (For Loved Ones)

completely stymied by the parking meter. With my non-functioning brain I had no idea how to use the machine to get a ticket. While tears continued to stream down my face I asked a young lady for assistance. Looking at me strangely, she explained and finally, with shaking hands, I managed to get my Visa card into the slot provided.

Karen, the Social Worker, met me in the Emergency and led me to a Family Room. "They are stabilizing him and then he'll be going for a CT scan. I'll let you know when you can see him. A doctor will come and speak to you and let you know the extent of his injuries. Are other family members coming?"

Unable to speak, I could only nod.

With no one to talk to, my only company was the terrifying images that plagued my thoughts. I could not control my flood of tears and no matter how many times I brushed them aside, they continued to fall. It was like trying to contain water in a bag made of cloth. The half hour or so I sat alone in that room with my brain alternating between mush and the horrible images that cascaded through my head, my usually calm nature did not hold up very well.

My youngest son was the first to arrive, having taken the rest of the day off work; another of my sons was the next to get there.

"You may see him now," Karen told us as she quietly rolled her wheelchair into the Family Room.

Confined herself to a wheelchair, she was the perfect person to be dealing with those in times of stress. She was the calm personality I had leaned on in that first hour or so as she periodically checked on me.

Knowing by now that Larry had hit and slid under a tractor mower, I was surprised and relieved that his face was not as I had imagined it might have been in that time while I sat alone. Road rash extended from his forehead and down his cheek on the right side of his face and on the left side he had another injury which was still heavily crusted with blood. Both eyes were badly bruised, particularly his left eye which was completely swollen shut. Although he was heavily medicated and appeared to be unaware of our presence, I whispered, "I love you," as I leaned over his hospital bed.

The doctor smiled sympathetically at us. "He was conscious when the paramedics arrived on the scene as well as when he arrived here although he's been very confused," he told me. "Because of his confusion, he's being taken for a CT scan to determine if there is any brain injury."

Someone interrupted soon after, "I'm sorry but you'll have to leave. We will be preparing him for surgery now."

Shortly after that Larry's youngest son arrived. He was very upset. He had nervously ridden his motorcycle to the hospital – the only transportation he had available. One of my daughters-in-law arrived shortly after that and only minutes later his daughter and grandson. Then my son, daughter-in-law and the baby from Chilliwack arrived with yet another son of mine. When Larry's son, daughter and grandson quickly went in to see him, my second son's girlfriend showed up, also having left work in order to be there.

It probably wasn't long but it seemed like hours before the emergency room doctor came out to talk to us. We were told he had broken both shoulders, his collar bone, had multiple rib fractures, both lungs had collapsed - now with drainage tubes in them; his skull was fractured with possible brain injury; some broken bones in his left hand and both legs were badly broken with his left knee particularly injured with loose bone fragments. "He'll be going up for surgery to his legs soon. It'll be about five to six hours before he'll be in ICU (Intensive Care Unit)," the orthopedic surgeon told me. He then had me sign a consent form allowing for a blood transfusion and the surgery.

Shortly after that my youngest son went to pick up his girlfriend and then my ex-husband arrived. Everyone was there except my daughter, the small grandchildren, my mother who hadn't as yet been told, and Larry's eldest son.

Someone from the emergency room staff gave me a bag with the clothes they had cut off him and the police woman gave me his effects (ring, watch, necklace and wallet). One of my daughters-in-law put these things in her car so I didn't have to deal with them.

Not knowing what to do after the police woman came and gave us a brief explanation of what she thought happened (she had not as yet spoken with any of the witnesses), we went up to the second floor where the ICU was while we waited to hear the results of Larry's surgery.

After having heard nothing for almost four hours, one of my daughters-in-law and I were finally able to stop a doctor in the hallway near the operating room and asked if he knew how much longer the surgery was going to take and how it was going.

"It's taking longer than they expected because of how extensive the injuries are to one of his legs," he told us. "It could possibly be another two to three hours."

My ex-husband then said he would take everyone for dinner at the Chinese restaurant across the street. We all went except for Larry's youngest son. Feeling sick to my stomach, I had to force myself to eat thinking that perhaps food might help the nausea. It didn't. The nausea remained.

When we got back to the hospital, Larry had just been taken to ICU from surgery but we still weren't allowed to see him. Eventually they said he could have a few visitors, two at a time only were allowed. One of my daughters-in-law and I went in first and then Larry's daughter and grandson.

A Roller Coaster Ride With Brain Injury (For Loved Ones)

"Who are all those people?" the Intensive Care nurse asked, a deep frown creasing her forehead.

"We're a very large family," I answered.

"Well I can't allow everyone in tonight," she told us gruffly.

As a result, only four of us got to see him on that first night. I stayed for another couple of hours, along with my eldest son and his wife and then we were told to go home.

"He's being looked after," she told me. "Right now you have to look after yourself. You won't do him any good if you get sick."

My eldest son and daughter-in-law suggested I stay at their place so I wouldn't have to be on my own and it was also closer to the hospital than our own place. My son drove me to our place to pick up some things rather than me driving on my own. I realized when we got back to the house that I had left the paint and the brush out. My son took care of that and whatever else that needed to be done. My brain still felt like mush and wasn't functioning at full capacity. Thoughts seemed to escape me before words could be spoken.

Arriving back at my son's place, they gave me a glass of wine to help me sleep but I slept not at all. How could I? It was our first day in Hell.

CHAPTER TWO

Life Has Changed

August 23

On the second day Larry's face was so swollen that he was barely recognizable. The bruising was worse. There was no response when I spoke to him, although when the nurse called loudly (they all speak loudly in ICU), his eyes fluttered open briefly. He was on a ventilator. He was having difficulty breathing on his own because of the extreme pain he was in from so many injuries, particularly the broken ribs. They had also put him on heavy doses of morphine in an effort to control the pain.

The doctor came and spoke to those of us who were there; myself, my eldest son and my daughter-in-law. "Larry is stabilized at the moment but the serious concerns now are infection, blood clots and pneumonia," he told us. "We've put him on antibiotics because he's developed a fever." (His fever continued for several days and a fan was at his head constantly in an attempt to help lower his high temperature).

In his first full day in ICU the nurse said that he was doing miraculously well. "I have seen people come in with fewer injuries than Larry has who haven't done as well as he is doing," she told me. That one comment buoyed my spirits beyond belief.

My daughter-in-law (my oldest son's wife) spent the entire first few days with me and for that I was extremely thankful and grateful. It was good to have the support and not be alone when I didn't know what was going to happen. The first couple of days I went to the hospital at 8:30 a.m. and stayed until 9:30 p.m. They were agonizingly long days. Larry was only allowed close family visitors at that time. During the first week or so, many in the family visited him almost every day, including one of my sons, his wife and their baby who made the long drive from Chilliwack each time.

August 24

At 8:30 a.m. on the third day, I was surprised to see that the bruising on Larry's eyelids was already beginning to fade but his face was still very swollen and his arms and legs were beginning to swell. They began therapy on his legs so that scar tissue wouldn't form to restrict the mobility of them. They said it would also help him with his circulation.

"You can stay if you like," the therapist told me."

Holding his hand, I felt his grip tighten when she began to bend and stretch his legs, particularly when she was working on his left leg which was the one that was most seriously injured. Watching him, I saw his face contort with pain, and feeling myself break out into a cold sweat, I put my forehead onto the cool railings beside his bed. But as she continued to work on his leg and his grip became tighter, I felt nausea begin to build up within me. I didn't realize that I had almost passed out until I felt the therapist help me into a chair. As I sat in the chair with a glass of cold water, I realized I would not be much help to him if I behaved like that. I did not stay for any further therapy sessions. I realized they did not need to be looking after me when their duty was to look after Larry.

The orthopedic surgeon came to check Larry and said his legs were healing well so far. He said that even his badly injured left knee was looking good and he didn't think Larry should have any problems with it in the future.

* * * * * * *

During the next few days, while Larry was in ICU, I went to the hospital early each day and continued to stay with my son and daughter-in-law. My daughter-in-law, bless her, continued to come for a large part of every day, to keep me company.

By the fourth and fifth days, the swelling on his face began to recede and the bruising was fading even more rapidly. I found I was now beginning to be able to stay in the room for longer periods of time without feeling nauseous or weepy. However, on the fifth day, while standing beside Larry's bed I again suddenly became so nauseous I had to leave his bedside.

On the sixth day, the nurses in ICU began to reduce the pressure on the respirator to encourage him to make an effort to begin breathing a little on his own. His fever also seemed to be subsiding somewhat. All of the medical staff worked hard to keep him as comfortable as possible by trying to manage his pain level and seemed to be pleased with the way he was coming along.

I went home for the first time, but because I didn't want to stay on my own, I invited my two grandchildren to stay at the house with me. In those early days, a girlfriend also stayed overnight several times. The support I received in that early period from family and friends helped me so much through this difficult period. I realized how fortunate I was to have so many wonderful people in my life.

CHAPTER THREE

Changes To Rejoice In

August 28

Until this time I hadn't had a chance to notify anyone other than family and the closest of friends so I began to send e-mails notifying everyone of Larry's accident. Trying to keep everyone apprised of his accident was impossible to be done by cell phone when I was spending almost all of my time at the hospital. (Cell phones had to be shut off while I was in ICU and standard phones were difficult to find in the hospital).

* * * * * * * * * *

The seventh day was the beginning of some very big and important changes for Larry: At this time he would briefly open his eyes if the nurses spoke in a very loud voice to him and a few times he moved his mouth in what seemed to be an effort to talk. He was having difficulty trying to speak because of the breathing tube, so what he tried to say was largely not understandable.

On this day I sent an e-mail to update family and friends:

'There has been an improvement in Larry's condition. He is having a few wakeful periods and this morning seemed more aware than he has been so far. He even attempted to smile at me although his eyes were open for no more than seconds at a time. Today they decreased the amount of air he is getting through the respirator so that he is breathing mostly on his own now. The amount of pain he's in because of his broken ribs and shoulders is what is holding him back from completely being able to breath on his own. They are going to try another pain killer that doesn't knock him out like the morphine does and they have also said they may use an epidural in his chest area to control the pain. Tomorrow they plan to remove his breathing tube completely – hopefully. Today they also removed the last drainage tube from his lungs which is another great improvement. He squeezes my hand and his grasp is quite strong. The bone surgeon said that he is healing nicely and he didn't expect he will have problems with his legs – he said even the knee that was so injured appears to be doing well. He said he will be in a wheelchair for two or three months and there will be a lot of therapy afterwards. The swelling in his face has gone down and the bruising is fading.

Tomorrow or the next day should bring several more big changes when they remove his breathing tube completely and begin to wean him off the morphine.

I will keep everyone posted as often as possible on his improvements. If anyone wants to phone for more info, I'm home later in the evenings – after 9:30 p.m. is probably best.'

I spent most of the days in ICU with Larry except when they asked me to leave for turnings, changing dressings, doctors' rounds or when procedures were being done on other patients.

However, on the eighth day, Larry had a nurse who was a very efficient, no nonsense kind of person. She only allowed me to stay with him for fifteen or twenty minutes at a time with at least an hour or more between visits. "He'll become overtired if you stay too long at a time and sleep deprivation can cause disorientation," she told me sternly.

During one of my fifteen minute sessions of sitting beside Larry, she reproached me with, "Please don't rub his arm. Quite often patients with brain injuries will become over stimulated and agitated."

My initial thought was that a patient knowing he had someone close by might possibly heal more quickly and feel better. When I suddenly realized she had said, 'brain injury', it stopped me short. Outside of when the doctor had initially mentioned the possibility of Larry having a brain injury, this was the first time it had been mentioned. It was the very beginning of my realization that his injuries were perhaps even more serious than what I had previously thought.

August 30

"What can we expect regarding Larry's recovery?" I asked his ICU nurse.

Looking at me over the top of her glasses she said, "Well it could take as long as a year, or he may never be the same."

"But he's strong and fit and very healthy," I told her.

Removing her glasses completely as if for emphasis she said, "But he's no spring chicken, you know."

On this day, they took Larry's respirator tube out and gave him an oxygen mask. Although he was not always obviously conscious or aware he sensed the feeding tube and oxygen mask and constantly tried to pull at them. Because of this, they tightened his restraints, but in his semi-conscious state he continued to struggle with them and still managed to pull the mask off and the feeding tube out of his mouth.

"It's very dangerous," I was told. "He could die if the fluid drips into his lungs unnoticed."

They then decided to put both the feeding tube and the oxygen tubes down his nose. The restraints were a continuous frustration to him, as were the tubes, and he fought constantly with them. In his more lucid moments, he tried to get any visitors he had to remove them.

I sent out another update to everyone on Larry's progress:

'Some more very good news. They have completely taken away the respirator; they then had an oxygen mask on him but now have only the little prongs in his nose. They took another tube out of his chest and now instead of five monitors, he only has two. His feeding tube is now in his nose so he is able to talk a little although I still can't make out most of what he says. He smiled a couple of times again today and he had his eyes open fairly often for brief moments. He must be feeling better because as he becomes more aware that he is restrained, he becomes more frustrated and wants me to untie his hands. He is not happy when I won't do it. They also had him sitting up on the side of the bed today for a few minutes. The nurse is trying to force him to do some things for himself. It's amazing what a difference there has been in the last two days. The nurse said the neurologist apparently doesn't think there will be any long lasting serious damage from his brain injury but it's difficult to say definitely this early, she said. I will keep you posted.'

He was becoming more aware, smiling several times at me and once he gently stroked the side of my face. Another time he motioned me closer and I thought he was going to say something but instead it felt as if he had kissed me on the cheek. He had been making some effort to talk but became very frustrated with his difficulty at being understood.

I asked one of the ICU nurses about his brain injury because, outside of it being mentioned that he had a brain injury, no one had given me any further information. She said the neurologist said it didn't appear that it was severe but they really wouldn't know the extent of it until he was up and around, talking and functioning.

August 31

On the tenth day there was another big change. He was moved into the Critical Care Unit (CCU). He was also beginning to have longer periods of wakefulness.

They had asked me to leave when they moved him to CCU and when they let me back into the room, the nurse said, "Look who's here. Do you know who this is, Larry?"

Looking at me he answered, "Steve."

"He's just joking," I laughed. I soon realized however that none of his answers were making any sense. It wasn't long before I became aware, with a sick feeling of dread in the pit of my stomach that he probably hadn't been joking and maybe he didn't really know who I was.

Later in the visit, he began to look at me very strangely.

"Do you know what my name is?" I asked him.

With a puzzled look on his face he said, "It isn't what you want it to be."

"What do you think I want it to be?"

"Coffee and toast," he answered.

When my son and his fiancé came a short time later I asked, "Do you know who they are?"

Looking at my son he said, "Pseudonym."

"Pseudonym?" I asked.

Smiling at me, as if he had a private joke he wasn't sharing, he said, "He has an alibi."

After some disjointed conversation he told them that there was going to be a meeting at the rail at 8:30 tomorrow morning and they had to be there. It was very important. He became quite agitated that they might be late for the meeting.

In a panic I asked, "Can you name your children?" He refused to answer me.

Having moved to a new home two months previous to his accident, I asked, "Do you remember the new house?"

He had no memory of the new home and in asking questions I quickly realized that he appeared to have very little memory of anything prior to the accident. My son's fiancé began to cry and I felt like I was going to throw up. The move to CCU seemed to have totally disoriented him.

Quickly finding a nurse I tearfully said, "He doesn't seem to remember anything from before his accident. Is he going to get his memory back?"

"It's his brain injury. We have been asking him dates and he has no idea what month it is or even what year it is. He thinks it's 1996. He's had a very serious bump to the head. We'll just have to take it one day at a time. If he continues to be disoriented," she added, "they will probably send him for another CT scan."

'How would he know me?' I thought. 'We didn't know each other in 1996.'

It was my first real awareness that Larry's brain injury was likely to have a very serious impact on our lives. I was suddenly faced with a new reality.

As a result of the move to CCU, Larry's pain was particularly severe and also increased when they tried to get him to do more therapy. When they attempted to loosen the phlegm in his chest it caused him considerable pain so they were forced to increase his morphine dosage in an attempt to control his pain level. Unable to use their normal methods for breaking up the phlegm because of his multiple rib fractures, they sat him up to suction out his chest. As a result, his blood pressure soared to high levels as he violently fought the procedure.

CHAPTER FOUR

Panic Sets In

September 1

On the eleventh day, Larry was as confused as he had been on the previous day. He had no idea where he was, even though he had been told repeatedly that he was at Royal Columbian Hospital.

I again spoke with the nurses who told me they didn't know when his memories would return. "There has been some shearing of his brain. He's also had contusions (bruises) which were caused by the force of the impact."

(From my research):

(This type of injury drives the brain against the bony ridges inside the skull. When this happens, small blood vessels (hematomas) are broken, causing bleeding. The bleeding can occur between the skull and brain (epidural or subdural hematomas) or inside the substance of the brain (intracerebral hematomas). If they are sufficiently large, they will compress the brain.)

Larry's injury caused damage to his frontal lobe. Fortunately, it appeared as if his were smaller bleedings which the medical staff seemed confident would eventually be absorbed into his system. (In spite of the fact that neither the bleeding nor the swelling appeared to be extensive, shearing results in the death of neurons.) They could give me no definite answer with regard to the severity of his brain injury at this time.

I brought pictures in of the family to try and jog his memory. Some people he seemed to vaguely remember while others he didn't at all. *I didn't realize until much later that part of the problem may have been that he wasn't wearing his glasses and some of the pictures were possibly too small for him to see. (I had given him his glasses but he emphatically insisted that they were not his and he couldn't see with them).*

September 2

I sent out another e-mail to keep everyone posted on Larry's progress:

'Physically, Larry is coming along well. His breathing tube is out, he is talking and he's getting stronger. Today he sat in a chair for a few minutes. He doesn't appear to be in as much pain or at least he's not grimacing with every movement like he has been previously. He is still getting a little bit of oxygen and he still has a feeding tube in his nose which he hates. He is now in CCU. They have said that he will be going up to a ward when a bed comes available. That is the good news. The bad news is that his brain injury seems to be much more extensive than what they had originally led me to believe. I don't understand because he wasn't in a coma, (except for the medically-induced coma). I thought he had no extensive bleeding and apparently no extensive swelling but the attending nurse in CCU said that he got such a bang to his head that his brain has been sheared. Larry thinks it's 1996. He knows some people but not others. One person came in that he has known for twenty-five years and he did not recognize him. The nurse said hopefully he will get his memories back. That is all they are saying.

"As for visitors to CCU, I'm not sure who they allow. I will keep you posted.'

While Larry was in CCU, he always smiled when I came into the room as if he knew me even though if it was 1996 as he insisted it was, we had not as yet met. Most times when I asked what my name was, he said it was Sylvia. On other occasions, he wouldn't answer.

I asked him different questions to try and jog his memory. A few things he remembered, but most things he didn't.

* * * * * * * *

During this time, he often seemed to be very agitated and almost constantly seemed to be looking for things: his tape measure, a pen, his business cards which he wanted me to give to the nurse (that damn Brit, he called him), another time for a knife and fork (he was still on intravenous), once for coffee and another time for his cell phone.

"Who do you want to phone?" I asked him.

"Sylvia," he answered.

"You can tell me," I told him.

"No I can't."

"Why?"

"Because it's private and a secret."

His behavior was very child-like and he kept trying to be funny, as children will do. After he said what he considered was his little joke he would look to me as if for approval and then roll his eyes. Through all of his maneuverings he never ceased struggling with his restraints and his continuous efforts at trying to pull his tubes out.

* * * * * * *

Over the next few days, as various people came in, there were a few he recognized but many he didn't. There seemed to be no rhyme or reason as to why he recognized some and not others, at least not with regards to the amount of time he had known them. I went over things we had done and places we had gone with him in an effort to try and jog his memory.

"Do you remember our trip to Mexico?" I asked one day.

"No. Tell me about it."

Mentioning a few things like our visit to Virginia City and some of the people we met in San

A Roller Coaster Ride With Brain Injury (For Loved Ones)

Felippe, he occasionally was able to add a few memories of his own.

"And do you remember looking for covered bridges?"

He smiled and said, "And we found some too."

"Do you know who this is?" I asked when one of my brothers came in.

He remembered my brother's last name but didn't remember his first name, giving him the name of 'Scott' when in fact his name is 'Dennis'.

Sometimes he would stare at the wall and when I asked what he was looking at would say things like: "'Franklin' or 'wheels and keys'". He stared at the ceiling a lot too and wanted to fix it. The ceiling really seemed to bother him.

One time he asked, "Are you ready?"

"For what?"

"We've got to get some lumber."

"For the garage?" I asked, surprised that he had remembered the work he was going to do in the garage.

With a puzzled look, he said, "No, there's work around here that needs to be done."

He talked a lot about coffee and fish. One day when his daughter and grandson were there, he'd had a running conversation about a fish. When I was going to leave he said, "Take the fish with you."

"No, I'll leave it with you."

Then, when his daughter and grandson went to leave, he wanted them to take it too. When they didn't want it either, he got quite annoyed and said, "Well leave the damn fish then."

* * * * * * * * *

One day I was later than usual getting into the hospital. He seemed to be quite annoyed with me and barely acknowledged my presence when I got there. And then later when I wouldn't undo his restraints he said, "Why don't you get the f....k out of here." Although I didn't realize it at that moment, it was the beginning of his quite lengthy period of nastiness. There were other times however, when he seemed good natured and was very affectionate with me.

Because he couldn't remember much of his past, I tried doing memory exercises with him. Often he would stare at me and stubbornly resist doing them or else he would shrug and say nothing, completely ignoring my efforts at trying to help him with his memory.

At other times he could be quite funny and would roll his eyes after he had said something and had gotten a laugh.

I received many supportive e-mails from friends and, of course, family. The following is one from a friend:

'Sylvia, glad to hear Larry is coming along. Hope the confusion is clearing up. Drugs can take a long time to clear the system and we are all different in that regard.

"Are you at the hospital every day? Can I pop by and see you there? Maybe have a cup of coffee and hear how YOU are doing through all of this. Life sure takes its twists and turns – just when we think we have it all figured out.'

'Hi,' I answered. 'I am at the hospital every day but the last two days for only a few hours each day because I've had my daughter's children. She's been in the hospital. She had a Grand Mal seizure – there's rarely just a shovel full of crap; usually it comes by the full load. If it was for my garden, I'd be happy for the load but not now. Anyway, thankfully, she seems better.

I get conflicting things told to me with regards to Larry – I've been told that it's his brain injury and he may remember things or he may not. Then I've been told it could be the medication and the bruise to his brain which will take time to heal. I asked to speak with the neurologist but they said it was just a wait and see thing. By all means come

A Roller Coaster Ride With Brain Injury (For Loved Ones)

by; a break would be great. It's rather stressful when he says things that don't make sense. Thanks for keeping in touch.'

CHAPTER FIVE

In The Land Of The Confused

September 4

On the fourteenth day Larry got moved from CCU to the fourth floor orthopedic ward. However, when he got there he appeared to be even more confused than he had been previously and was extremely angry. (With each move he seemed to become further disoriented).

Around this time he also became aware of his bodily functions and even though he had a catheter, he was beginning to become very angry and agitated when he felt he had to go to the bathroom and there were visitors in the room. When I realized what the problem was, I asked him if he wanted people to leave the room. That appeared to solve the problem somewhat with regards to his agitation over that particular issue.

On the ward, Larry was assigned a sitter so one of his hands could be unrestrained but he became so violent with her that they were forced to totally restrain him again. While trying to get out of bed he glared and bared his teeth at her and said, "I have to frigging get out of here." When he started to get like that with me, I tried stroking his arm and saying 'sh-sh-sh, it'll be okay". Sometimes he would gradually settle down but, at other times, he directed the same type of anger towards me as well.

During those times, I left the room until he settled down.

He had a few visitors on the day of the move to the ward – my brother and sister-in-law (who he doesn't see often and who had just returned from Mexico), had come by. He didn't appear to recognize them. Also, one of my sons and daughter-in-law came in, as well as two friends. The friends brought a picnic lunch with them. I took a half hour and joined them up on the roof for a picnic. The sun was shining and it was a welcome break. Quite often, friends, after their visit with Larry, would take me out for dinner, dropping me back off at the hospital for my evening visit with him. I was extremely grateful for my friends and family during this difficult period.

He was now in a room where three of the four people were confused but the difference was that they were all in their 80's.

Larry continued during this time to talk about fish, fishing boats, smokehouses (none of which are or ever have been significant in his life). He talked about Indians on a front lawn in Edmonton getting together for a meeting and an idea for a movie where everyone was a dessert. He also talked a lot about petitions and meetings and tried to organize his visitors to attend various meetings.

A Roller Coaster Ride With Brain Injury (For Loved Ones)

September 5

The neurosurgeon, to my great relief, came in to see him today. "Do you know what month it is?" he asked.

"It's the month before next spring."

"Do you know what day it is?"

"It's the week after last Friday."

"Do you know what year it is?" Larry stubbornly refused to answer.

He was still very confused but slept for a good part of the day because most of the room had been awake for the better part of the night. One started acting up, then another and, before long, the whole room of confused people was awake.

I took pictures and albums into the hospital and things from home, as well as pictures of the new house, to try to help Larry with his memory. Some things he seemed to vaguely remember but other things not at all. I had the feeling though that he was getting tired of being asked, 'Do you remember?' and was agreeing in some instances without there really being a memory.

September 6

On the sixteenth day they removed his catheter and he again pulled his feeding tube out.

They decided to try the 'swallow test' on him. Fortunately, he was able to swallow.

It was another big step - two and a half weeks after his accident he was able to start on pureed foods and liquids. I'm sure he enjoyed the first solids he had tasted in more than two weeks. They continued with his intravenous although he still constantly tried to pull that out.

Another e-mail update regarding Larry:

'More improvement with Larry. He is no longer solely on intravenous. He was in a wheelchair for about one and a half hours today. He is getting uncomfortable lying in bed and is becoming bored as well. He is also still extremely confused.

In the early part of each day he seems to do better with regards to memory and doesn't go off on tangents as easily but later in the day his conversation is sometimes difficult to understand and follow as to content, not speech. He's got a good sense of humor although there have been a couple of the sitter/nurses he has taken a definite dislike to and has glared and bared his teeth at them. I talked to the neurosurgeon who said Larry has some fluid around the brain that usually gets absorbed into the body but he didn't anticipate there would be a need for surgery. He feels Larry is going to be fine but is just confused right now. (This was not a surprise to me). Larry still believes that it is 1996 and still has many areas where he has no memory. Also, his short term memory is almost non-existent in that he can't remember what he had for a meal eaten an hour previously and he doesn't remember any visitors after they have left. He's beginning to make connections with the people he recognizes, i.e.: my brother with golf and he mentioned the name of my brother's grandson who he doesn't see often. Previously it was difficult to know if he had made the connection between people. I think he has done fantastically well in two and a half weeks especially considering the extent of his injuries.'

Larry is still very frustrated and angry with bathroom issues and is refusing to use the bedpan. As a result he's becoming constipated. "It's like sitting in a cardboard box. My butt touches the bottom," he complained. One time when I gave him the urinal bottle to use, he looked at me with a mixture of fear and shock in his eyes and asked, "Do you expect me to sit on that?"

I wrote a poem entitled the Bedpan Blues thinking he might look at the situation with some humor.

> Patience please give me as I sit and wait here,
> The bedpan is coming, I face it with fear.
> A cardboard box I'm made to sit in,
> It feels like cement or ice cold tin.
> I sit and sit but the deed's hard to do,
> I don't want to sit here I want to be in the loo.
> Then pitted prunes they tell me to eat,
> And when I won't eat them they turn up the 'heat',
> With ex-lax and softeners they make me take,

And they claim that it's all for my sake.
I've only one wish and they say I must wait,
It's the loo that I want and the bedpan I hate.

He saw no humor in my attempt at poetry. Reality was too close, I guess.

During this time Larry was quite insistent on several occasions that he wanted to visit the 'Pope'. I thought this very strange because he is not a religious person. "Why do you want to visit the Pope?" I asked. I got no answer because there was none he could give.

He told me much later when he was no longer confused that visiting the 'Pope' is a term used for going to the bathroom.

September 7

On the seventeenth day there was a marked improvement in that Larry seemed more aware; and was quite talkative and bright. They had him sitting up on the side of the bed and said he would soon be ready to go for longer walks in the wheelchair. It wouldn't be quite so boring for him when he could see more than just the one small room.

On this day, as an experiment to see where he was in his 'memory' department, I reminded him of our 'welcome to our new home' party we were going to have. I asked him who we should invite thinking this might help jog his memory. In this list he mentioned some old friends that he had rarely kept in contact with in the last good number of years. When I mentioned some of the joint friends that we associate with regularly and suggested them, he just shrugged and said, "Maybe. I'm not sure if they'd fit in."

Larry was determined that he could get out of bed and the reasons why he couldn't had to be explained to him each time he tried.

He was quite cranky later in the day. I was feeding him his dinner and then he suddenly turned to me and said, "Why don't you get out of here."

"I think I will go," I agreed, reluctant to put up with his nastiness. "I'll see you tomorrow."

September 8

I took Larry for a walk around the hospital in his wheelchair so he could get a different view of his surroundings. He didn't seem to particularly enjoy the change and insisted on returning to his room after a short time.

He went off on a several tangents during my visit. At one time he thought one of his friends had something to do with raising me. When one of the nurses asked him questions relating to his health, he told her he had quit smoking three years ago but later he was looking all over for cigarettes. Another time, he looked at me with shock and asked, "Where are they?"

"Where are what?"

"Our drinks. I just poured them."

Then he was talking about some people who were riding in the arena. I later found out it was people he knew when he had been in his teens and had worked at the race track feeding and exercising the horses.

September 9

I picked up a squishy ball which I thought might help him with his arm and shoulder strength and also took a radio into the hospital that I thought may help relieve the boredom. He wasn't interested in either. I had also picked up a coffee at Tim Hortons since he had been so fixated on coffee but he wasn't interested in that either. In fact he wasn't particularly interested in seeing me either. He and all of the others in the room had been up for most of the night. He still didn't remember the new house and had no interest in looking at pictures of it.

I again decided to do a list, with his help, for our 'welcome to our new home' party to see who he would invite this time. On the list was a couple whose names were completely unfamiliar. When I again mentioned friends that we see often he said, "That won't work because the money is coming from the barbeque and the stairs."

When I asked him what year it was he said, "I think '86 or maybe '96."

I left shortly after I had helped him with his dinner because he was extremely cranky and nasty when he was awake and the rest of the time he slept.

September 10

Larry now has a male sitter with whom he seems to get along quite well. It will be very good for him, especially since he's in a room with eighty plus year old women who are as confused as he is.

"He knew what year it was today," the sitter greeted me. This was the first time he had been able to identify the year. That was a big step.

An e-mail received from a friend on September 10, 2006:

'We dropped in at the hospital tonight to see Larry. He was sleeping when we got there. I went downstairs and when I got back he was talking to Tom. He sure looks better. He said everyone is telling him that. He did seem to be quite disoriented though. I don't think he knew who Tom was but seemed to know who I was. He did mention about Norm coming in last night but for most of our visit he wasn't making sense. He seemed to have a good sense of humor and we had a few chuckles. We're thinking of you.'

And my response:

'Glad you got in to see Larry last night. It was my Mom's and one of my son's combined birthday dinner so I left earlier from the hospital than I usually do. He looks almost like his old self except that he's lost weight. Earlier in the day he was quite funny too although he kept insisting that he could get up. When I told him early in the day about the birthday dinner, he thought he could come along and couldn't understand why he couldn't. I told him maybe he'll be home by Thanksgiving. When I told him it was four weeks away, he became very angry. He was more aware and seemed to be more lucid today. Yesterday however was a very bad day. I was so depressed after spending the day with him that I invited my friend Maggie over for the evening because she's always a great cheerer upper. He doesn't do 'tired' very well. He was very cranky with me. He was better today and he even said he remembered a little about the new house. The sitter/nurse also said today was the first time he's known what year it is. I think he now knows who people are most of the time but he can't always put a name to them. I will talk to you soon.'

(From my research)

When there has been injury to the frontal lobe, there can be emotional and personality changes. Some of these changes can be due to the brain injured person's reactions and adjustment to the injury. Their frustration can cause anger which may sometimes be excessive. There may also be a "blunted affect" where they may be insensitive and unable to recognize what someone else may be feeling. They may become more self-centered in their feelings and behavior and they may be child-like in their behavior.

A Roller Coaster Ride With Brain Injury (For Loved Ones)

This was definitely the case with Larry. He appeared to have no awareness or concern when he said hurtful things to me or to others.

Before Larry's accident, he occasionally sneaked a smoke but since his accident he had not mentioned smoking. He had not mentioned drinking either although prior to his accident, he drank three or four stiff drinks of rye most evenings. Now coffee seemed to be the big thing. One day when my brother came to visit, Larry said, "I drink about six cups of coffee a day and then I go for the hard stuff."

"What's the 'hard stuff,' my brother asked?

"That's when I have it with cream and sugar."

* * * * * * * * * * *

Most days I asked if he knew what my name was and he mostly would answer my name although occasionally he would say something that didn't make sense and a couple of times he said my name was 'loverly' and 'cherishable'.

Another time I asked him, "Do you know how old you are?" but he fell asleep trying to think about it.

When he woke up I told him how old he was. After thinking about it for a few minutes, he said, "It doesn't sound as bad as I thought it would."

September 11

On the twenty-first day, he seemed less confused; he knew some of his visitors and he behaved rather well except for throwing some of his vegetables at the patient across from him. He also thought she was a man. When I told him he had been quite cranky with me a few days previously, he seemed surprised and rubbed my face and said he would "always be patient with me." (Unfortunately that was not the case for most of his hospital stay).

A friend called to say how upset he was with how disoriented Larry was when he visited him and in the next breath said, "Don't let it get you down." I was finding it difficult not to but I was fairly optimistic about the future. We just had to get through our 'todays, I knew.

A therapist gave Larry an assessment and although he did well in some areas, in others he did not. Memory was one of them. She said she would leave some cognitive exercises for me as I was determined to do as much work as possible with him. Through my research I discovered that the earlier cognitive exercises are begun after an injury, the more successful the prognosis was found to be. Telling Larry what I had read, I said, "When we are doing these cognitive exercises I would like you to be patient with me and I will be patient with you."

I brought an album in and as I pointed to pictures of friends and family, he did very well. It was the first real improvement I saw regarding his memory. And he didn't go off on too many tangents.

He fell asleep shortly after dinner and I left to meet two friends for a walk on the beach. My friends and I had a late dinner while we watched the sun go down. It was a perfect way to unwind with the support of friends, a beautiful sunset and the sound of the waves washing up on the beach.

September 12

Larry seemed to be in good spirits when I got to the hospital. I was anxious to get him started on cognitive exercises as soon as possible. It had been devastating to discover that the cognitive therapist was off on maternity leave and had not been replaced. I discussed how I felt about this with the therapist who did the assessments and thankfully, she was quite willing to get me all the exercise sheets that he would have been given to work on had there been a therapist available. With this material I would be able to work with him myself. It may have been a God-send actually because as a result of me having the material readily available he probably would get more one on one than if we had relied on a therapist entirely.

Some days he was completely resistant to doing any exercises, but other days he was fairly willing. On the days he was completely resistant to doing them, and there were many, I tried to explain that if he didn't do therapy he could have problems that may very well last him for the rest of his life. "And," I said, "they won't be just your problems, they'll be other people's problems too."

We worked on them for a couple of months and I could see the improvements as we progressed. What he wasn't able to do one day, two or three weeks later he was better able to try and often completed. I believe very strongly that these therapy exercises helped him immensely. I wonder how many patients with brain injuries 'slip through the cracks' if they don't have this material or someone able to help them on a consistent basis?

** Samples of some of the Exercises I did with Larry are at the end of this book.

A doctor came and spoke to me, asking what I thought as far as Larry's confusion and memory were concerned. "I think he's improved a little over the last couple of days," I told him.

"That's good to know. We want to get a base line of his cognitive abilities. He had quite a bit of bleeding in his brain but we're expecting that it will be absorbed into his system. Depending on how he does, he may get transferred to Queen's Park Therapy Centre in New Westminster for follow-up therapy, although if he does really well he may be discharged from here. He'll be here for a while though anyway."

Today Larry remembered one couple who had come in before I got to the hospital. This was good but he also mentioned that a second couple had come in as well. The sitter said only the one couple had come in.

In the afternoon Larry thought he was at Home Depot. He went off on a few tangents and when I was going to leave, he insisted that he was going to come also.

"But you can't," I said.

"If I can't go, then you can't either," he insisted.

"But I can't stay here."

In a huff he turned his back on me, quickly falling asleep. I left while the getting was good.

September 14

Larry was very confused today and went off on a lot of tangents. He thought he was skiing in Whistler with the brother of a friend of his. This particular friend doesn't have a brother but he had a name for him anyway. And he thought the friend's wife was his sister. These are people he has known for thirty-five years or so.

"But you don't ski," I reminded him, "and you hate the cold weather. Why are you skiing in Whistler?" He just looked at me with a puzzled expression on his face.

Because he seemed to be so confused I asked him several times during the day if he knew my name and each time he did. When I asked, he was quite adamant that he didn't want to do any cognitive exercises. As the day progressed he became crankier and when I decided to leave, he again said, indignantly, "Without me?"

"Larry, I have to go. You can't come with me. You have to stay here."

Glaring at me and almost hissing he said, "I am not staying here another night even if I have to stay at the hotel next door."

"You'll feel just as uncomfortable in a hotel. They're looking after you here. They won't in a hotel."

Still glaring he declared stubbornly, "I'm not staying."

I went to talk to the nurse to tell them about his behavior and when I returned, he had fallen asleep, so I left. He never seemed to remember the following day that I had left him when he hadn't wanted me to go.

I had been impressed with the hospital staff and their concern for the patients. I did, however feel that communication was not what I had expected it to be. I found that unless I tracked down the appropriate people and asked questions in order to get the answers I needed, no one approached me with information – not the doctors, the neurosurgeon or the therapists. I did find though, that when I asked they were approachable and my concerns were addressed as soon as possible. The web sites relating to brain injuries that the librarian of the hospital library e-mailed to me proved to be extremely helpful, although even with those, there was considerable 'weeding through' to get the answers I needed to my questions.

To further complicate things, getting differing opinions and answers from various professionals on Larry's care was confusing, i.e.: *How should things be done? When would he be ready for therapy? What type of therapy would he be able to do?*

Then there was the question of whether he would be discharged to Queen's Park Care Centre, GF Strong or home. Because I was often told differing things by different staff members, I was never sure what to expect from one day to the next. Looking back, the confusion may have resulted from the fact that no one ever seemed to be entirely sure of the extent of Larry's brain injury or of his prognosis.

I became aware that, as time went on and the more hours Larry spent awake and the more tired he became, the more likely he was to go off on 'tangents'. One day he insisted for most of the time I was there that he had been at a railway station with a friend of his.

Another time he thought he'd spent the day over on the Island and one day he thought he was on the Sunshine Coast.

He was very often insistent that we had to get out of there. "I'm afraid you can't go anywhere.

You have to stay in the hospital until you get better," I'd tell him patiently.

"If I can't leave then you can't either," was his usual answer, often becoming so angry with me that he'd turn his back on me, eventually falling asleep.

When he became particularly difficult, I would speak with the nurses. "With brain injuries it is three steps forward and two steps back," they would tell me.

Many times it felt like two steps forward and three steps back.

September 15

"I was stealing dogs last night," he told me when I arrived at the hospital. "It's a dog like Jeremy has."

"But Jeremy" (his grandson) "doesn't have a dog," I reminded him.

"What happened to it?" he asked in amazement.

"He's never had a dog."

Deciding to change the subject, he then said he'd been stealing cars and the dogs were in the car. Then looking at me he said, "It wasn't very nice that the police woke us up at 7:00 a.m. this morning to take us for breakfast. I heard them in the living room calling us."

A Roller Coaster Ride With Brain Injury (For Loved Ones)

The doctor said Larry would be going for another CT scan in about a week when I voiced my concern regarding his continued confusion. "We'll know better then. I suspect that he will need extensive therapy. His recovery could take a few months or it could be a couple of years. He may never be the same. We just don't know right now."

I talked later in the day to another friend who had been in to visit Larry and he said Larry had thought he had delivered the friend's son and that I was in the bed next to him.

September 16

Most days I asked various questions trying to revive his memory. "What kind of car do you drive?" I asked him today.

"A 67 Olds Cutlass," he answered. In actual fact he drives a '95 Blazer. Another time he told me he drove a black Panther.

There were some good days but there were a lot of bad days. On the bad days he was confused, going off on tangents and often very difficult and cranky but almost always confused.

One day he had gone down for x-rays and, knowing this, I asked how his morning had been.

"There was a little guy who wanted to take pictures of me and he wanted to be in some of the pictures with me. But when I looked on the walls, there were pictures of this guy all over the place."

On another day when I went to the hospital he was surprised to see me. Why are you surprised to see me? Didn't you think I would be in today? I'm here every day."

"I thought you had gone to Africa with Chris. A few people have asked about you and I told them that's where you'd gone. 'There's going to be a lot of surprised people when they see you," he told me.

Over a week or two I had noticed Larry had been flirting with the nurses and making inappropriate and suggestive remarks to them. "I've heard Larry say rather inappropriate and suggestive remarks to the nurses. Will he continue to do this?" I asked the doctor.

"The frontal lobe of his brain has been affected and injury to that area affects judgment," he explained. "It is fairly common with patients who have had frontal lobe injuries to behave inappropriately in this way."

Deciding to talk to Larry about it, I told him it was embarrassing for the nurses and it was also embarrassing to me when he behaved like that. "Are you aware that you say inappropriate things?" I asked him.

"As soon as it's out of my mouth I know," he answered.

I later told the occupational assessment therapist that I had talked to him about his inappropriate remarks. She said it was a good thing to make him aware of it. My conversation with him seemed to have gotten through to him because I didn't see that behavior after our conversation unless he was just being more careful in my presence.

(From my research):

Frontal lobe injuries involve planning, organizing, problem solving, selective attention and inattentiveness, personality, behavior disorders, emotions, memory, judgment, inhibitions (lack thereof), elaboration of thought, impairment of recent memory, social behavior, impulse control, difficulty in interpreting feedback from the environment and often personalities can change significantly.

Larry's frontal lobe brain injury appeared at this time to be moderate in severity.

(From my research):

One of the symptoms of moderate brain injury is confusion for sometimes days and/or weeks. There are usually physical, cognitive and/or behavioral impairments which can last for months or may be permanent. However with treatment those with moderate brain injury are usually able to make a complete recovery or successfully learn to compensate for their deficits.

Behavioral Symptoms include mood swings, denial, inability to cope, difficulty with emotional control and anger management, difficulty relating to others, agitation, delusions, paranoia and sexual dysfunction.

Cognitive Symptoms include impairments of perception, communication, reasoning, problem solving, planning, sequencing and judgment, lack of motivation and inability to initiate activities.

September 16

Friends came to visit Larry today and we were looking through the album of our trip to Mexico. He did very well, adding some memories of his own of the trip. He even remembered which side of the garage I park my car in at the new house and told them that he was closing in the carport.

Because he was doing so well, after they left I asked him if he remembered some of the stories he's been telling. Laughing, he said he did.

"They're all fantasy. Do you know when you're making them up?" I asked him.

"Yes, it's like when the Indian chief....." and he embarked on another fantasy story.

"I was golfing last night," he later told me seriously.

"You were here."

"That's not what the guys who were with me said," he declared as he glared at me.

"Those are more fantasies, aren't they?" I asked him.

"I want to get out of here," he said in an effort to change the subject.

"Remember," I reminded him, "you can't go until the doctor gives you the green light. It's not up to me to say when you can leave."

He backed off and didn't pursue the argument.

An e-mail from a friend and my response – September 18th:

'Thank you so much for remembering our anniversary when you have so many other things going on. Hope every day is improving for Larry. Remember to drop by any time.'

'Maybe I'll try to drop by tonight on my way home if that's okay. Larry was doing quite well yesterday. He didn't seem to be quite as confused as he was on Friday. On Saturday I asked him a lot of questions and he did well and didn't go off on too many tangents. I took my grandson, Reilly in for a visit yesterday but after carrying 43 pounds of him from the parking lot, with his cast on, up two flights of stairs, along with Larry's housecoat, two bags of cars and a train to keep a young boy amused and my heavy purse, I was really regretting my decision. Thankfully there was a wheelchair at the door in the Emergency that I could put him in. I was glad I did though because Reilly had Larry laughing and for the most part he seemed quite lucid.'

An e-mail sent to everyone about Thanksgiving Dinner on September 18, 2006:

'Hi Everyone, I'm going to have Thanksgiving here on Monday, October 9th. I've already got the turkey. I will put the turkey in the oven and then visit Larry and if everyone could bring something that would be great. Larry was very confused on Thursday and Friday (after they had increased his pain meds). I mentioned it to the nurses and they took him off the extra one and on Saturday and Sunday he was much better than he had been – he said the occasional thing that was off but his memory seemed to be pretty good.

Today he seemed to remember a few extra things on his own. He did go off on a few tangents again but he still has fluid and blood around his brain which would account for that. But there definitely is an improvement. I hope everyone can make it.'

September 19

I picked up a Burger King hamburger and milkshake for Larry. He ate and drank half of each and I ate and drank the other half. He was extremely cranky – not particularly at me – he just was. After an hour, I was ready to leave.

"I think I'll go home after you have your lunch," I told him. He gave me a dirty look, rolled over and fell asleep. I stayed because I didn't want to sneak away without saying goodbye to him.

When he woke up about an hour later he was in a better mood although he was more confused and went off on several tangents. He seemed to be more lucid with some of his visitors, not necessarily the ones he's known the longest, (perhaps he makes more of an effort with those he doesn't know as well).

The doctor came in again today. "Larry will need a lot of cognitive therapy and they will be sending him to a therapy clinic for rehabilitation. A cognitive therapist will see him to determine what his requirements will be and will place him on a waiting list," he told me.

CHAPTER SIX

Doing Things His Way

September 20

Today, thirty days after his accident, I arrived at the hospital and was told by his nurse that Larry had gotten out of bed and walked to the bathroom. He was not supposed to bear weight on one leg for eight weeks and on the other leg for twelve weeks. In his right leg he has a pin from his knee to his ankle running down the centre of his tibia and held in place with screws. In his left leg he has a plate holding his femur together with screws attaching the plate to the bone and screws holding the pieces of bone together in his knee.

"You know, Larry," the nurse explained, "you could injure yourself and end up having to spend more time in the hospital than you may otherwise have to. If you re-break your leg you'll be back at square one again. The bone has to heal around the plate."

Larry agreed that he didn't want to be in the hospital longer than he had to be. I thought that was the end of the matter and presumably so did the nurses.

A few days later Larry was again caught walking – down the hall – with his bare butt hanging out of the back of his night shirt. This is the man who was too embarrassed to be seen wearing shorts in the summer because he thought his legs were too thin. The nurse again said, "If the bone isn't given a chance to heal around the plate and the rod, it will require another operation. You're doing yourself damage. "

But Larry was convinced that he can walk and insists he can go to the bathroom on his own. He won't listen to the nurses, the doctor or to me. "We'll just negotiate the time I have to stay off my leg," he told me.

"Larry," I said with a fair amount of exasperation, "some things can be negotiated but the healing of bones can't be; it is one of those things that just have to be accepted. The healing process can't be hurried but it can be hindered and it definitely can't be negotiated."

"Everything can be negotiated," he told me angrily.

They sent him for x-rays and decided that, as yet he hadn't done any extensive damage. After his last escapade they put a monitor on his bed so that if he tries for another adventure, it will alert them. He was extremely angry about the monitor.

"I wasn't walking in the hall," he later told me belligerently. "I was up on the roof and no one said anything about that. I spent the night up there and then they left me sitting in a wheelchair all morning. I met Todd at the railway station too and no one worried about that either." (He doesn't know a Todd).

He was becoming an increasingly difficult patient. One of the nurses told me it was for this reason that he wouldn't be going home because of how difficult he would be for me to handle. "You're wrecking it for yourself," I told him. "If you don't listen and you don't do as you're told, you'll be staying in here a lot longer."

His only answer was an angry glare.

September 21

Larry was very frustrated when I arrived at the hospital today. He said he had wakened later than usual and everyone had gone and he was alone. He said he had wanted to talk to a doctor about getting out of there but they didn't know what he was talking about. "Then," he said, "they took me downstairs and did some x-rays on my chest but they didn't know what they were doing down there either. One person said one thing and another person said something else. Then they were looking for you and no one knew where you were." He glared at me as if everything was my fault.

"I have a job that has to be done on the Sunshine Coast but how can I when no one knows what they're doing?"

"Maybe you were having a dream," I suggested.

He looked at me with shock. "I can't very well put that in my quote now, can I?"

The cognitive therapist did another assessment to compare it with the previous one. "He's done much better than last time," she told me.

"When am I going to come home?" He asked me yet again.

"The therapist said they wouldn't send you home yet because you would be too difficult for me to look after. They've given me some more exercises to do with you. If you do them, it might help."

He continued to argue with me when I tried to get him to do the cognitive exercises. And he still wasn't sure where he was. When the nurse asked him earlier in the day he told her he was in Surrey Hospital. When I asked later, he said he was in Vancouver General Hospital.

I again asked him to help me make up a guest list for our "welcome to our new home" party. It was my continuing experiment to see how he was progressing. This list turned out to be typical of what our guest list is like including close friends and the whole family. I could see him mentally making an effort to go through our phone book and he included almost everyone we would normally invite to the party. This was a fantastic new improvement in his development over his last two lists. I was very optimistic when we had completed it and was very glad that I had begun this experiment to chart his progress.

September 25

When I got to the hospital Larry again seemed surprised to see me. Other than that, he seemed to be fairly lucid. He did, however, continue to complain about having to stay in the hospital and about having to use the bedpan. When I asked him how he felt he said like a piece of cotton batting – weak, useless and blah. He said that emotionally he was one step up from how he feels physically but from what I've seen, it's probably not a very big step. He said feeling frustrated covers most of it. The last three days have been fairly good. I tried another poem for him:

I Want To Go Home

Why don't they listen to me when I say,
Get me out of this bed, don't make me lay,
So many long weeks they've forced me to stay.
I want to go home and I want to go now,
If they won't let me, I'll make a big row.
I really won't walk if I can go home,
I'll really be good and will not roam.
Stand on my feet, I will not do,
If I don't listen I know I will rue,
The day that I didn't listen to you.

Larry was no more impressed with this one than he had been with the Bedpan Blues.

September 26

An e-mail from a friend:

'We just got back from the hospital. We had a wonderful visit with Larry. What a difference! I guess everything just takes time.'

And my response:

'When I got to the hospital and asked if anyone had been in, he said you had which was great because now he's starting to show some short-term memory. He also said his sister had been in and then later he said it was someone else so I'm not so sure about that one. He also remembered that the doctor had been in to see him in the morning and sure enough when I talked to the nurse, she said that another cognitive assessment had been done on him but she didn't have the results in the file yet. He said that the doctor said they would be moving him to another place (which is true because they've told me that too). He also remembered being told about how long it will be before he can weight bear. I knew but hadn't told him because I didn't want to discourage him with the length of time and I certainly didn't want to be the messenger. He was pretty cranky about that and said he would go crazy. He fell asleep and when he woke up he was in a better frame of mind but he had remembered he had been cranky before he went to sleep so there is a huge improvement today and in fact, improvements in the last few days as far as being confused. Yesterday and the day before, we did a lot of work on the exercises and he did very well. He didn't want to work on them today though. I'm glad your visit was good and that you saw the improvements too.'

A Roller Coaster Ride With Brain Injury (For Loved Ones)

September 27

When I got to the hospital Larry said he had been asking for a telephone since 6:00 a.m. so he could phone to tell me what is going on. He said he was getting frustrated and bored. He said he's the last one to get his breakfast in the morning and they help everyone before they help him. The biggest problem is he doesn't feel well because he's constipated and he doesn't want to use the bedpan.

I suggested that we do exercises and he again refused.

"It's very important that you do them every day so that your brain is stimulated. We want to repair the damage and it's important to begin as soon after the injury as possible. You don't want to have any life-long problems, do you?"

He wasn't convinced so I got my book and decided to read instead of talking to him.

"Okay," he finally said, "two pages."

"Three," I said.

"Okay," he reluctantly agreed.

Two friends came in and were very impressed with the improvements they saw in Larry today since they had last been into the hospital.

September 22

On the thirty-second day however, there was suddenly an awareness and insight into his confusion. "You have been very confused," I said to him on that day. Have you realized when you've been confused?"

"Sometimes," he told me. "I notice the expression on people's faces when I've said something that doesn't make sense; then I realize that something isn't right. And when you've asked me questions and I think about the answer but what comes out of my mouth isn't what I had thought in my head. It even sounds strange to me."

Shortly after Larry's sudden new awareness, he began to become very critical of everything, i.e.: he didn't like any of the food; they were late with it; they were too early with it; didn't they know what they were doing in x-rays? He didn't want to use the bedpan; they didn't bring the bedpan when he needed it; they left it too long; he couldn't use the bathroom; they wouldn't bring the commode; they brought the commode but they didn't put it in the bathroom; and on and on the litany of complaints went. On one of these days by 1:30 in the afternoon, I was looking at my watch, willing away the hours so I could go home.

September 28

An e-mail sent to everyone with an update on Larry's progress:

'I am very happy to let everyone know that Larry is doing very well. The last four days or so,

A Roller Coaster Ride With Brain Injury (For Loved Ones)

most of his confusion seems to have disappeared and when he occasionally says something that's from out in left field, I can quickly get him to focus back into reality. He now knows when he says something that doesn't make sense and he said that even he wonders where it has come from but it doesn't happen as often now. And it's great that he has that awareness. I have been working with him on exercises almost every day to stimulate his brain – some days he is more reluctant to do it than others but he's doing well at the ones he has done so far. Of course now that he is feeling better he is getting frustrated and bored so I brought him some different kinds of crossword puzzles, etc. and his clip board and paper and I'll pick up the Province and hopefully something in it will jump out at him and tick him off so that he'll want to write some letters to the editor. He likes doing that and I think it would be a good exercise. They caught him walking again (I know this sounds wonderful – it is (in that he can walk) but it isn't because he's not supposed to put any weight on his legs for some time yet. They had to take x-rays again to make sure he hadn't injured his legs. He is now monitored in bed. He's not happy about that. His memory is completely back even for little odds and ends of things right up to the time of the accident. His short term memory has been bad even to the point that in the afternoon he can't remember anything from the morning. But the last two days he has been able to remember a few things that have happened in the morning by dinnertime and this evening he even remembered who came in last evening so there's a big improvement there too. Today he was moved from the acute care room (across from the nurses' station) to down the hall to a convalescent room because he doesn't require as much care now. He is now waiting for a bed at a rehabilitation centre where he will get therapy. But with all the exercises that I have been doing with him (and I don't think I'm being unrealistically optimistic), I think he's been doing amazingly well with them and it really hasn't been that long (only three weeks if you only count the time he wasn't heavily sedated). Several people have been in the last couple of days and they said we're getting the old Larry back – they've seen such an improvement in just several days.'

Larry was moved into a room with three other men which, I believe, was a God-send for him. (To this day he remembers nothing about the accident and for almost five weeks after but from the time of this move he has some memory of a few things).

After his move, he was back to his old tricks of getting out of bed and back to the bathroom he went. He was again caught and put on a very state-of-the-art monitor system this time. After that if he sneezed, they knew it. Of course he was very angry about the new monitor and insisted vehemently that he could be trusted even though he continually proved to everyone that he couldn't be.

He still continued to be somewhat resistant to doing the cognitive therapy exercises. And I still insisted that they needed to be done or he may never get well. He usually did them but it was rarely without a fight. I also got him a book of

Suduko puzzles that I thought he might like to try as well as the crossword puzzles he always has done.

He still kept insisting that if he had to stay in the hospital, he'd leave. "No one is telling me what I have to do."

"Unfortunately," I told him, "they can tell you. You have to be patient. You have to heal."

"I don't know if I can be patient," he grumbled during one of these discussions.

"You really have no choice but to be patient. You have to do what you can to help your legs heal by not damaging them. And you have to help your brain by doing the exercises. It's your body and you have to be proactive in your own health care. Other people are willing to help you so you should be willing to help yourself."

He was so frustrated and angry that I really got nowhere with this line of reasoning.

The neurologist came in to see him and said he was doing much better than he had expected him to be doing right now. Larry felt good after talking to him and so did I.

September 30

An e-mail from a friend:

A Roller Coaster Ride With Brain Injury (For Loved Ones)

'Larry's progress is so thrilling. The brain is an amazing organ. I had to laugh when you talked about giving Larry the Province – hoping something would tick him off so he'd get busy letter writing! I just know you are the best person in the world to see Larry through these next months of recovery...stimulating him in the ways that will keep him engaged with life outside the four walls of his room. You are going to be pretty intensely involved in his care giving for months to come...so please let me know when you want to take some time out for yourself to go out for coffee or lunch. I'd love to see you.'

My response:

'Ironically after I wrote that e-mail to everyone, he didn't do as well. He got into a wheelchair on his own in the morning and went to the bathroom – these are no-no's. He was tired and didn't have a good night so he had a little more problem with confusion, frustration, etc. I will call on you when he is doing therapy. Right now I feel that since he isn't getting any at the hospital and he's so frustrated I am going to try and do as much as I can in that area – whether he wants to or not because obviously I want his success to be as good as it can be. It should be done as early as possible and they don't have a cognitive therapist at this time. The down-side with me doing it is that he will say 'no' to me but probably wouldn't to someone else.

Today I decided to sleep in – some friends are down from Westbank staying here for the weekend so I will be going in later than I normally do. And yes, once he's in a regular rehab program, I will take some time for myself and I would love to get together.'

When I went into the hospital and tried to get him to do his exercises, it was another argument. I explained what the possible repercussions were for not doing them but I got nowhere. Later in the day he did finally agree to work on a couple of pages.

"The doctors aren't telling me anything," he continued with another one of his ongoing rants.

"They are and so have I. I've told you the situation several times a day for the last few days. You can't put weight on your legs. It's a wait thing and you can't hurry the healing. You just have to be patient."

"I don't know if I can be."

"You have no choice but to be patient." I repeated the same thing over and over, hoping that he would understand.

Finally he agreed that he would be but I know that promise would last only until I was out of the room if not sooner.

An e-mail to a friend – October 3rd:

'Thanks again for dinner and the lovely evening. I enjoyed myself although I was probably more tired than I've been since the very beginning of this whole thing.

On Sunday Larry was the most difficult he has been to date. Nothing pleased him. He argued and disagreed with everything. Previous to that he had refused for about three days to do any of his mental exercises.

Yesterday, thank goodness, he was in a better frame of mind. I told him how difficult he had been and that I didn't need to be talked to in the way he was speaking. He said he hadn't liked himself too much on Sunday either. I tried to explain to him he was making the situation worse for himself than it had to be when he behaved that way. I was told that they're holding off on sending him to Queen's Park Care Center also because of his behavior. They don't have enough staff to look after patients who are difficult to handle like he is.'

Answer from friend:

'I guess anger is part of the healing process but unfortunately he is aiming it at you. I think it is normal. Maybe he needs someone to talk to him – man-to-man.

Or maybe a counselor if one is available. Sounds like it's time for a glass of wine, why don't you stop by tonight?'

My response:

'I know it is common to react with anger to the ones who are closest to them and I'm not surprised even though I was frustrated. I've talked to the social worker and mentioned his behavior but I didn't suggest that perhaps a counselor could talk to him. I've tried to get across to him that I know it's frustrating and it seems a long time but there is no alternative that won't harm him and hinder the healing process. If he doesn't accept what he has to do, he will make things more difficult for himself and in the grand scheme of things, he will look back and think it wasn't such a long time after all when he's alive and doing well. He might have had to accept a lot worse fate than twelve weeks or so in the hospital. One doctor said he's very lucky that he has all of his limbs.

Thanks for the invitation but I'm behind on things that I really have to do. I'll talk to you soon.'

Unfortunately Larry is not only being difficult with me but he's making it very difficult for the nursing staff. I asked them if he was possibly depressed which was my opinion but I don't know if it was ever followed up on. At any rate they gave him no medication for depression.

When I went in I told Larry how difficult he had been the day before. He made an attempt to be reasonable because when I suggested doing the cognitive exercises, he agreed without an argument; he didn't complain during our walk; he didn't try to get out of bed; and he didn't make an issue about not being able to go into the bathroom. He was much more pleasant so I stayed longer than I had during the last several days.

On the forty-first day after his accident, Larry had an opportunity to go to a restaurant across the street for a retirement dinner with myself and a group of people we know. Initially he seemed to be excited at the prospect but on that day he decided he wasn't going to go. "I'm not going to go to a banquet hall with my bare butt hanging out," he told me angrily.

"It won't be. You'll have pajama bottoms on, a shirt and a jacket and a blanket across your knees. We have walked around with you wearing much less than that."

"I told you, I'm not going in that toilet chair," he said referring to the commode chair.

"It's not going to be in that chair; it'll be the wheelchair."

Looking at me angrily he said, "That's not what you told me last night. I won't be able to go to the bathroom if I go in the wheelchair."

"That's why I think it's a good idea to go to the bathroom now. Then you won't have to worry about having to go when you're there."

He continued to go round and round with his arguments, emphasizing the fact that he didn't want to go with his bare butt hanging out. Then changing the subject, he started on his usual argument. "I'm not going to stay here. Everyone else comes in and has an operation and can leave but I can't." Telling him that they have different types of injuries was not getting through to him.

He then began his other recurring tangent which was that no one tells him anything.

"Yes they do Larry," I repeated as I had so often previously. "The nurses do, the doctor does and so do I. You're just not remembering." But the whole conversation, as with many of his tangents, went nowhere.

The end result was that I went to the retirement dinner on my own. (They had decided to have it at that restaurant so that we would be able to attend). I decided that I was not going to allow him to spoil it for me. And I was not going to stay and listen to his long list of complaints.

Over the next few days he again continued to resist doing any exercises for his brain injury. Instead he continued to whine, complain and in general be difficult. His continuing poor behavior came as a complete surprise to me. This was a Larry so unlike the Larry I had known before his accident. However, from doing research on brain injuries, I had come to realize that this behavior is indicative of the injury he had sustained. Unfortunately, knowing this in theory and dealing with the situation in real life are two completely different matters. Being optimistic by nature, I continued to have a strong belief that he would get better.

I began to wonder again whether Larry was depressed and spoke to both the social worker and the head nurse. "He insists that white is black and is completely unreasonable most of the time; he argues about everything and doesn't listen and then insists no one is telling him anything." (I realize now in hindsight that I should have followed up on this with more diligence because he did not receive medication for depression).

He continued to complain about the monitor being on his bed. "It wouldn't be there if they could trust you not to get out of bed and put weight on your legs."

"That's not the reason. It would be on there anyway," he responded. But he couldn't give me another reason why it would be on.

One day as I was leaving Larry asked me what I was going to be doing the next day. "I'm picking up Reilly and looking after him for the morning, dropping Nick at school, making phone calls to people about how things are going with you, doing things that need to be done around the house, and then I'm coming to visit you probably about 12:30 or 1:00."

"It must be nice to just do what you want to do and then come here for a nice visit."

The irony of his comment had me laughing. He didn't see the humor. I usually stay until about 6:30 p.m. or 7:00 p.m. with an hour drive each way;

go home, get dinner and try to get a few more things done.

This, I also discovered through research, is also very indicative of people with brain injuries; they tend to feel sorry for themselves and can't see anyone else's position at all. They also often may have difficulty recognizing their own deficits and their impact on others.

While he was in the room with the three other men, they were giving him a bad time about wearing a beanie helmet when he was riding his motorcycle. He defended it by saying there wasn't anything wrong with his head and it wouldn't have helped his legs and his other broken bones if he had been wearing a full helmet. (Logic was not a strong point with him at this time).

CHAPTER SEVEN

Changes On His Road To Rehabilitation

October 4

On day forty-four Larry had another big move. After gathering up his things at Royal Columbian Hospital, I said thank you and good bye to the very nice staff there and met him at Queen's Park Care Centre, his new residence.

The new facility he'd been moved to was a nice, bright cheerful hospital with very friendly staff. I told the nurses about his tendency to get out of bed so they also put a monitor on his bed there. He was not happy with either me or the staff.

An e-mail to everyone – an update on Larry's progress:

'Good news. Larry was moved today from Royal Columbian Hospital over to Queen's Park Care Centre which is a rehabilitative care centre where he will be getting therapy. They took him there by ambulance and he was pleased about the move. He's been very frustrated lately about the sitting and waiting so now things will hopefully start to be done. They are going to continue to monitor his bed though because he still doesn't realize the importance of not putting weight on his legs. He thinks that a quick trip to the bathroom isn't going to do his legs any harm.'

Larry's mood and disposition didn't improve with this latest move and a couple of times when I was visiting he asked me to leave, usually accompanied by a fierce glare.

"This will either strengthen our relationship," I often found myself thinking as I drove home with tears running down my face, "or it'll break it." How it could possibly strengthen it though, I did not know.

Shortly after Larry arrived at Queen's Park Care Centre, a neurologist came in and spoke with him and did an assessment. "It will be Larry's head injury that will keep him in the hospital longer," he told me.

At Queen's Park Care Centre, Larry seemed to become even more frustrated and angry. He became a very difficult patient and he began 'lumping' me in with those he considered were the 'bad guys' (the hospital staff). Trying to get him to do any exercises to help with his memory and other issues with his brain injury was like butting my head against the wall. During this period of time, he thought the staff should be doing things for him and he shouldn't have to do anything for himself even when he was able to.

I reminded him of the ball I had brought in previously so he could squeeze it to build up the strength in his hands and upper body- he wouldn't do it. I brought in another type of 'squeezie' thing and he wouldn't use that either. I again suggested that he be proactive – that it's his body and he should have the most interest in making it well. He insisted that it wasn't up to him; that they should be doing things with him to build up his strength.

There were also four television viewing areas but he wouldn't use any of them. Even after he'd gotten over a super bug he developed he continued to stay in his room. He talked to no one. He told his visitors that he had been told he couldn't go out of his room. When I asked the nurses, I discovered this was not the case.

However, this latest move seemed to help as far as his confusion was concerned. He still had occasional lapses but I began to think it was more that he was having difficulty with his day to day memory. Each day when I came into the hospital I asked him what he could remember of the previous day and of the morning before I got there. He remembered very little; not even who had been in to visit him either before I'd arrived or after I'd left the day before. Not all days were bad; some were better than others.

He had breakfast brought to him but was expected to go to the dining room, completely dressed, for lunch and dinner. At no time that Larry was at Queen's Park did he comply with this and he made no effort to interact with any of the other patients. He went once to an exercise class and decided he didn't like it so he refused to go again. He insisted they should be taking him to the exercise pool but they couldn't because he couldn't weight bear and he wouldn't listen to instructions and/or couldn't remember them. He refused to understand when told the reason. He argued about taking showers and for the most part, he refused except when I occasionally was able to convince him. He also saw no need to put on clean pajamas on a daily basis. In short, he was a very difficult patient.

October 4th – 20th

I asked one of his nurses about his therapy. She said that because he was unable to weight bear, she wasn't sure what type of exercises they would be doing with him.

"What about his upper body and his brain injury?" I asked.

She didn't know anything about his brain injury. I hoped I was not going to continue to be his 'only' cognitive therapist. The physio also didn't get in to see him and I couldn't talk to the doctor because he was only in on Mondays, Wednesdays and Fridays early in the morning so, in the beginning, I always missed him.

During this period Larry often asked me to leave. Because I was saying the same things (i.e. not to put weight on his legs, etc.) as the nursing staff, he considered me to be part of the 'enemy'. Some days he was so difficult that I dreaded having to go in again the following day.

A Roller Coaster Ride With Brain Injury (For Loved Ones)

An E-Mail to a friend:

'Larry is now able to do the transfer to the wheelchair on his own and is able to use his right leg to pivot and weight bear (not walk on) so he can now get to the bathroom on his own. (If he had stayed at RCH, (Royal Columbian Hospital), because it is mainly a trauma hospital, I think it would have taken him awhile to get to this stage). AND they have given him a day pass to come home for Thanksgiving dinner now that he can do this. He's pretty excited about that prospect. The physiotherapist seems to be really great. He talked to us and answered a lot of questions after he went over Larry's file. The nurses are all very nice and helpful – even asking me if I want coffee or ice cream. Larry now has his own room. Talk to you soon.'

The day pass for our family Thanksgiving dinner was Larry's first time out of hospital since his accident. I had prepared dinner and then left to pick him up. My mother came to oversee everything while I was gone. There were going to be eighteen of us for dinner.

The dinner went quite well, with only one episode of confusion. He insisted that he'd had a glass of red wine at someone's house a couple of weeks ago. I reminded him that this was the first time he'd been out of hospital since his accident. He was adamant that he'd been out before and that he'd had a glass of red wine although he couldn't remember whose house it was. (I always tried to make him focus on reality instead of going along with what he thought 'reality' was). He ate well and seemed to enjoy himself although he was very quiet, not participating in much of the conversation.

My first attempt at getting Larry into my little Echo from his wheelchair was a challenge while I tried to keep him from weight bearing. Getting him out of the car and into the wheelchair was equally as difficult. At home, between three of us, we carried him and the wheelchair into the house.

An e-mail from a friend:

'How did Thanksgiving and Larry's first outing go? We were thinking of you two. How is Larry's rehabilitation going? It will be nice to see his progress.'

My response:

It went very well. I picked him up about 2:00 p.m. He did very well as far as sitting for such a long period of time. He did have to rest on the couch a couple of times for a short period of time but that was all. There were eighteen of us. He said even though he was very tired, he really enjoyed it. I didn't get him back until 9:45 p.m. I'm going to have the girls' birthday dinner on October 22nd so hopefully he'll be able to come home for that as well.

His physiotherapist is away until Monday and his doctor confirmed that they wouldn't start physio until he got back. I think part of the reason that physio has been rather slow is that he can't weight bear yet, only pivot which is what is helping him get into the wheelchair on his own now. In one week he'll be able to weight bear on the right leg and I'm sure that's what they're waiting for. But because he's so frustrated about having to wait, when I left the hospital tonight I asked the nurses if they could give him any kind of exercise to do so that he at least thinks he's starting on something to help his therapy progress. They said they were doing rounds tomorrow and they would discuss it at that time. I said any exercise at all would help his frame of mind.

Also the cognitive therapist doctor who saw him at Royal Columbian Hospital came in to see him again. He asked him some questions and did some exercises with him and said he did better than the last time he was tested. I think myself there's been some improvement even in the last week.

Larry fell out of bed today but thank goodness he landed on his butt and not on his legs or we'd have been starting from scratch again. He had been turning from sitting and unfortunately I didn't see what happened because I went to turn off the alarm. He said the bed moved when he turned but I may have moved it when I shut off the alarm. But the big and the small of it is the brake wasn't on and that is why the bed moved so easily. He was going to try to get back into bed by himself and I wouldn't let him. I called down the hall and two nurses came running to his room. They put him in some kind of contraption and hoisted him back up on the bed. Luckily he seemed to be fine in spite of his latest mishap.'

A Roller Coaster Ride With Brain Injury (For Loved Ones)

The physiotherapists assisted him in being able to use the walker since he could put weight on his right leg. After they had left his room he miserably insisted that it was a waste of time using the walker and he still couldn't understand why he couldn't begin therapy. He'd been told repeatedly that he had to wait until he could weight bear with both legs. He didn't agree with the doctor and nurses on this issue. They did, however finally take the monitor from his bed because it went off every time he got up to go to the bathroom. He was supposed to press the call button when he got up but he never did. I tried to explain that it was because they didn't want him to fall and hurt himself. He ignored my explanations. (Larry refused to recognize that since he had been in Queen's Park Care Centre, his mobility had increased by the fact that he was able to get in and out of the wheelchair by himself and was able to use the bathroom on his own and, had he wanted to, he could have made use of the recreational opportunities the care centre provided. He also was able to use the walker which provided him with much more mobility but he still didn't take advantage of using it to leave his room. I felt these extra aides to his mobility were definitely a therapy of sorts.

Around this time, when I was able to convince him to work on some of the cognitive therapy exercises again, there were questions where he was required to remember three things but was only able to remember two. That was an improvement over a few weeks earlier when he could only remember one thing and often had difficulty remembering the question almost as soon as it was asked. I showed him one exercise that he had tried to do three weeks previously. His previous effort at trying to do it hadn't made any sense to me whatsoever. Studying it himself, he said, "But that doesn't make any sense."

"Hallelujah," I thought. "We're finally making some progress here."

When he tried it again, he was able to do the exercise correctly. It was instances like that where I could really see the improvements he was slowly beginning to make. They were not daily ones I realized but they were being made weekly or semi-weekly and they were improvements nonetheless.

An e-mail from a friend:

'How are you doing? Is Larry still in Queen's Park? I am sure it will take a while for all the healing he will need. It is called one day at a time. Hoping all is going well for both of you.'

My response:

'Larry is frustrated and very cranky but he's now able to weight bear on the one leg and so he is able to use a walker. Supposedly he is to use his arms and shoulders so as not to put too much weight on his other leg. I think he's putting weight on it though. He has to get x-rays on his legs on Wednesday and then we'll see what the status is with regards to his left leg and whether or not he has been putting too much weight on it.

I was so frustrated with his behavior one day that I left. Most days I stayed for about six or seven hours but I left after only two hours. I was picking him up for a birthday dinner. He had been able to get a day pass for Thanksgiving dinner as well.

With regards to his brain injury, there had been no professional therapy done with him because the therapist in Royal Columbian Hospital was on maternity leave and was not replaced. But I was able to get exercise sheets from them. It's been an argument with him though the whole way along. His memory to the time of the accident is completely back but he doesn't remember anything from the day of the accident. The area that is his biggest difficulty is his short term memory. He can't seem to remember his recent 'yesterdays'. There are exercises for that as well which I'm trying to convince him are extremely important to do.'

By day fifty-five he was certainly becoming more aware of what he was saying and seemed to realize when he said something that wasn't right. He did still tend to make up stories from little bits he remembered hearing or by putting the little bits into the wrong context. And he was still having trouble with his 'yesterdays' such as not being able to remember conversations, etc.

About this time, the physiotherapist told Larry they would have to wait and see what the x-rays on his legs showed before they could let him do therapy on his legs. He also said that his brain injury was holding him back from getting therapy because of his memory problems in that he didn't remember instructions for exercises they gave him. Then one day he knew the day and date but he still couldn't remember where he was (Queens Park) or where he had been (Royal Columbian).

I had asked for several days to speak to the occupational/cognitive therapist. Apparently they were very short staffed so I didn't get to speak to anyone for a while. Eventually they did hire a part timer. She came in on her first day and got some background information and I asked her about things that Larry may be able to do and made some suggestions which she said she would run by her supervisor. She wanted Larry to get dressed to determine his level of self-care. He was successful in being able to do it on his own without putting his socks on his ears and his underwear on his head although I wouldn't have been surprised if he had thought that it would be a great little joke.

By this time I had finished with the exercises I'd received from the cognitive therapist at Royal Columbian and hadn't obtained any more from the therapist here. I was anxious to continue with mental exercises so went on the Internet to find more exercises that would be particularly good for the memory portion of his injury.

One of the suggestions I discovered on the Internet was to read a newspaper article to him and ask him what it was about in order to be able to determine what his comprehension level was like. He did fine with that. Another was to have him read and find different streets on a street map book. He did well with that exercise too.

There were also several exercises to help with his memory. One was to take an object, study it closely, thinking only of that object. After the object has been removed and some time had passed he was to either write down or tell someone everything he could recall about the object. The idea was that, as he became better with this exercise, he was to wait longer and/or find a more detailed object.

The second exercise was to write down everything that had happened and what he had done during the day including conversations and anything else that had happened.

Later in the evening he was to try and recall as much of the day as possible. As his memory improved, he was to wait until the next morning before recalling as much as he could. Larry refused to do both of these exercises.

CHAPTER EIGHT

Anger and Frustration

October 21

Day sixty-one was the beginning of some more new changes. Around this time Larry's frustration and anger were becoming very specifically directed at me. On this particular day when I got to the hospital he was cranky and complained about the therapist not knowing what she was doing; about them doing nothing for him; how he had to sit and twiddle his thumbs all day watching the sun come up and the sun go down; that he hadn't gone for a walk today; and that now they were putting cream on his feet and legs for no reason.

"We're doing it because you have a fungus," one nurse told him patiently as she liberally spread the cream onto his legs and feet.

Shrugging he said, "Well, knock your socks off then."

When I asked him if he had practiced his memory exercises, he brusquely answered "No".

"Have you practiced with the ball?"

"No," was his immediate and irritated response. "Why should I have to do it, they're the ones who are supposed to give me therapy?" He continued to complain about them not letting him put weight on his leg. "If they really cared whether I put weight on my leg or not they wouldn't have given me a day pass."

"They're hoping that you're not going to – that you're going to do what you're supposed to do." (It was understandable that he was frustrated about not being able to do things but he was not helping himself; he wouldn't listen when he was told he had to be patient and that his leg had to heal.) He was so bad tempered with me that I left after only two hours and sadly had to admit that I could hardly wait to get out of the hospital.

On the following day, Sunday, Larry had a day pass. I had previously prepared some of the dishes for dinner and Mom came over to oversee everything for the 'girls' (my three daughters-in-law) birthday dinner while I left to go and pick him up. When I arrived he was still in his pajamas. He hardly said a word to me as he got dressed. With his continued silence, I wheeled him out to the car and helped him into it. After we had driven for a little while, he still hadn't said anything. I tried to make conversation by saying which route I was going to take and with each thing I said, he made no comment.

I drove a while longer and finally asked, "Are you going to sit there the whole time without saying anything?"

"I tried," he said, "but I got no comment."

I didn't understand what he was doing – transference or something – because I was the only one who had spoken until that point and he was the only one who had made no comment.

After we got to the house, with so many people around, he finally began to talk. I later discovered, however, that he had been sneaking liquor and had poured himself three drinks of rum; undoubtedly very strong.

When I took him back to the hospital he said, "I'm sorry. I do appreciate everything you do." He very slightly redeemed himself at that point; but only slightly.

A couple of days later I asked Larry if he was surprised when I had left on the Saturday. "No," he answered, "I wish I could have left myself too."

That same week Larry went for x-rays. "Good news," he greeted me with when I arrived at the hospital. "I can't weight bear for four more weeks but the doctor said I can probably go home next week."

My heart almost stopped beating at the prospect of bringing him home. I wasn't ready for him to come home while he was in his present state of mind. I didn't know if I could hold up to twenty-four hours of nasty treatment and being talked to like I was nothing more than a rat in his garbage.

"But I can't watch you twenty-four hours a day to make sure you don't injure your leg. You can't be trusted not to put your weight on it. If you could guarantee me that you would do as you are supposed to do and wouldn't be nasty to me, it would be a different story." (The comment about going home was made by the orthopedic surgeon who had no idea what his behavior had been like; he had been speaking from a surgery point of view).

"I can't guarantee you that," he told me.

"Have you thought about how your behavior and how you are treating me is affecting our relationship?" (I realize as I write this that it was a ridiculous question. At that point in his recovery, our relationship was the least important thing to him. This is one of the symptoms of frontal lobe brain injury; i.e.: being self-centered and having little realization or concern for how another is feeling).

Refusing to answer my question, he repeated that he was not going to stay in the hospital for another four weeks. "Everyone around here seems to be more concerned about you than they are about me." He continued to be argumentative, unreasonable, sulky, self-centered and complaining. His nasty treatment of me was becoming increasingly difficult to handle and I spent most of each day either in tears or near to tears. His only response was to look at me with a look as if to say, 'What's your problem? I'm the one in the hospital.' All of the cognitive therapy I had been trying to do with him came to a crashing standstill.

A Roller Coaster Ride With Brain Injury (For Loved Ones)

The ICBC coordinator and therapist came into the hospital to speak with Larry and I and the decision was made to do an assessment on the house regarding railings and ramps. After they left, Larry angrily said, "They are NOT putting ramps and railings in the house." Then he sat and sulked and when I asked him what he was thinking about, he said, "I'm going to get out of this hospital, get my car insured, pick up some of my things and get a place near the clinic."

"You can't drive."

He glared at me and insisted that he could.

After about an hour of listening to him grumble and feeling the sharp edge of his bad temper, I'd had enough. My patience was beginning to run at a steady low. "I'm going to go now, Larry," I told him. "I'm not going to be your 'kicking post'. I don't deserve this treatment," I tried to keep the tears from sliding down my cheeks.

He refused to answer me.

"Don't you realize that you're making things difficult for yourself? This whole thing has altered my life too and it hasn't been easy for me either," I said.

He continued to ignore me so I left.

CHAPTER NINE

Looking After Myself

For the first time in sixty-six days I didn't visit Larry. I did however give the assistant occupational/cognitive therapist, a call. I told her about the previous day's behavior. "I am not going to let him take his anger and frustration out on me," I told her through my tears.

"You shouldn't have to allow it," she told me kindly.

October 26th – an e-mail to a friend:

'I didn't go to the hospital today but I did phone the assistant occupational/cognitive therapist. I've talked to her a few times before so she's aware of the situation but wasn't aware of his most recent behavior. I asked if there was a counselor who could talk to Larry. She said she will talk to the male therapist and have him talk to Larry and she would talk to him also. He needs someone else to talk to him, I think; not just me. She said he seemed to be down today. It will be interesting to see what his attitude will be like tomorrow. I hope it has improved. When I told her what has been happening and that I had left, she said, 'good for you'. She also said by approaching them and letting them know what's going on is keeping them on their toes.

A Roller Coaster Ride With Brain Injury (For Loved Ones)

I spent the afternoon doing more research on brain injuries. From the information I got, Larry appears to fall into the moderate degree level of injury. It said that those patients usually completely recover or, with adaptations, are able to adjust to their deficits. That was good to know. I have been pleased with his improvements but I'm afraid that his attitude and frustrations may inhibit his recovery. I know that frustration and anger are part of the behavior of people with multiple injuries and those who also have brain injuries. They are often not reasonable and they can behave inappropriately with regards to their emotions, particularly when it's the frontal lobe. He has to learn where to direct his frustrations and I know I'm not going to allow it to be directed at me. His attitude and behavior towards me have really been bad. He's insisting that he's going home or he will go crazy and he said he will start throwing nurses out the window if he has to stay there any longer. If he comes home now, I will go crazy.

He also seems to be very indignant that the staff seems to be more concerned about me than they are about him. I told him that I have a problem with him being home. I said if he did what he was supposed to do and wasn't nasty to me, it would be different. But he's proven that he can do neither. He agreed that he can't promise me. I told him if he insists on going home under these conditions, he's risking our relationship. He said he'll leave even if it means he has to stay at a motel. Since he's not supposed to walk this would be a difficult undertaking.

He has been completely unreasonable, negative, argumentative, complaining and disagreeable to me and he's refusing to do any more memory therapy or any upper body exercises. He said it's not his job, it's theirs. I said if he makes the effort, he would be proactive and it will do him good – that it would be for his own benefit.

There now, I'm whining. Sorry about that.'

Answer from the same friend:

'You were wise to leave. I think people may forget that it is not only difficult on the patient but also for the caregiver. You need some release from his foolishness. He has to realize that it isn't your fault and you have no control over the circumstances. He doesn't seem to be thinking rationally at all. I had hoped that he would start talking to other patients. You are wise to know that it would be impossible to have him at home under the present situation. It's too bad that he doesn't realize how fortunate he is to have you caring for him and keeping him company during the day. Don't apologize, you are not whining. I think you have been so supportive towards Larry. You need a break from the stress.'

On the following day when I went to the hospital, his eyes were bloodshot and he appeared to be a little teary-eyed. "I didn't expect to see you today," he told me.

"Why?" I asked.

"Because of yesterday and the other day," he answered.

I breathed a sigh of relief that he seemed to be aware of what his behavior was doing but it was only momentary. In minutes he proceeded to complain again about everything and everybody and how they had done nothing for him and he was no further ahead than he had been two months ago, etc.

Biting my tongue, I didn't ask him if he had done any of his memory exercises or upper body exercises. What would have been the use?

But I couldn't help saying, "Maybe things wouldn't seem so bad if you did something other than just lie here and feel sorry for yourself. Your attitude is not helping you with anyone around here."

"I know my attitude stinks but getting out of here is the thing that's most important to me right now. I'll have to see what happens after that."

"Is there anyone you like right now?"

After some thought he said, "I guess not."

I watched Larry as he lay in his hospital bed, a virtual stranger; he had changed so drastically since his accident. I sat silently, upset, and said nothing. I tried to think what could be done. Suddenly I thought that if he couldn't remember common sense things that got mentioned to him on a regular basis because of his memory difficulties, I would write everything down for him so that he could refer to them at various times during the day.

I made a list reminding him of the consequences of putting weight on his leg; on how he was making things difficult for himself by behaving the way he was with the staff; the consequences of not doing his memory and upper body exercises; and the risk to our relationship because of his behavior. He read it; put it down and then reread it.

"What do you think?" I asked hopefully.

He didn't answer for awhile and then replied, "You're right but I don't think our relationship needs much effort."

"It didn't used to," I said, "but it certainly does now."

"It's my leg that's coming between us," he said after some thought.

"No Larry, it's your attitude."

He was quiet for a while and when he finally spoke again he had lost some of his belligerence so the rest of the visit was a little more pleasant. When I went to leave he said, "There's a good guy in here, you know."

"I know that," I said. "Why don't you let him out?"

As I drove out of the parking lot that day, he waved to me from his window – weight bearing on both legs.

The following day when I arrived at the hospital, his behavior and attitude were a complete turn-around from the previous few days. He didn't whine, complain or argue. On a couple of occasions he started to say something, looked at me and then stopped, raised his eyebrow and said, "Sorry." He talked positively and made an attempt to be pleasant and cheerful and to carry on a regular conversation. He couldn't remember the memory exercises so I wrote those down for him also. It was a very pleasant visit – the most enjoyable we'd had for some time.

They also gave him crutches to use, cautioning him not to weight bear on his left leg. They decided to take his walker away from him because they could see that he was weight bearing. He of course, denied that he was. They said that with the crutches it wouldn't be as easy for him to pretend he's not putting weight on his left leg.

The ICBC therapist came out to do an assessment of the house. While we were talking she said, "I don't know if anyone has told either you or Larry but it is standard that when people have brain injuries their driver's licenses are taken away for usually a minimum of at least six months."

"I don't want to be the one to tell him that." I hadn't thought of that issue but realized when she said it that it should have been common sense.

"No, you won't have to. The doctor will be talking to him about it. Also when people have had brain injuries, it isn't advisable for them to drink alcohol, especially when there has been a shearing of the brain. It impedes the healing process and should be refrained from for a minimum of two years."

"And I definitely don't want to be the one to tell him that," I told her. "He's not going to be very happy about either of them."

"The doctor will tell him. Also smoking is a detriment. Smoking restricts the oxygen that gets to the brain and slows the healing process also."

'Poor Larry,' I thought, 'he's in for a whole lot of shocks.'

The following day when I went to the hospital I asked Larry if he had gone to the 'exercise classes' that the physio had told us about.

"No," he answered, "it's just a voluntary thing and it's not going to do anything anyway; I don't need it for my arms; I need it for my legs."

"How did your memory exercises go?"

"I didn't do them. I was thinking about it but I didn't. That Quack came in and said I can't drive for six months because of my brain injury," he fumed.

"You probably wouldn't be able to also because of your broken legs and because you can't weight bear."

"I am not going to go home and have you continually telling me that I can't weight bear on my legs. If that is what is going to happen, I'll go to a hotel," he glared at me.

"I won't," I answered. "You know you're not supposed to weight bear and you know the repercussions if you damage your leg; that you could end up back in the hospital. But if you do, I will not be coming to visit you every day as I have been doing. You'll be on your own."

After that conversation, most of his anger at being told he couldn't drive for six months seemed to be transferred to me (no doubt instigated by my comments). He spent the next few hours either being angry at me or sulking. Finally I decided that, brain injury or not, I was not going to allow him to talk to me the way he had been so I got him some ice and juice, put them on his table and left without another word.

The following day I made the decision not to visit Larry again, feeling it was too stressful and upsetting for me. During the previous weeks, because I was getting so stressed, I was beginning to feel that neither one of us was benefiting from my visits.

Calling the male therapist, I told him of my concerns regarding Larry. Because Larry seemed to respect the therapist, I felt perhaps he might be able to help defuse some of the anger. I mentioned his anger about being told that he couldn't drive; about his threats of going to a motel; how he seemed to have reverted back to a 'teenage mentality behavior' of not doing anything he was supposed to and not caring what the consequences of his actions were. I also mentioned that I'd noticed his general reasoning abilities, when it involved him personally, seemed to be off kilter, i.e.: he twisted conversations around that he had heard into what he wanted to hear; he said he'd move into a motel irrespective of whether he had a caregiver or not; he continually said that he knew he couldn't put weight on his leg or he'd be back in the hospital for fifteen more weeks and then he proceeded to do so. I also asked the therapist about the Acquired Brain Injury Program. He felt that Larry would be a good candidate for it.

"I'm more worried about his brain injury than about his legs. I know he's going to walk again," I said.

"We're all worried about that. We're also concerned about his behavior and how you are going to be able to handle him when he gets home," he told me.

I was extremely worried about that myself.

November 3, 2006 was the worst day to date. It was the day after the second day I didn't go in to visit him. Thankfully, a friend was there when I arrived and witnessed his behavior. He greeted me with, "The doctor said I can leave here tomorrow."

"That's not actually what he said Larry," our friend said.

Becoming nasty and belligerent, Larry insisted that was what the doctor had said. "And I'm getting a two day pass this weekend," he informed me.

"Did they approve it?" I asked, surprised that approval had been given with nothing being said to me.

"I told them. I'm coming home to put the railings up."

"How are you going to put the railings up when you're not supposed to put weight on your leg?"

"Watch me. I can do it without putting weight on my leg. They were supposed to have done them already. And when I come home, I won't be coming back."

"The therapist didn't come to do the assessment until this Tuesday and they're going to put them in next week. They won't let you leave if they know you're going to do that."

With that, he turned so much anger on me that finally our friend asked if I would walk to the elevator with her. "You poor thing, you look so tired. I feel so sorry for you," she said when we were outside of his room. "How are you going to handle him at home? I'd be afraid that he would get violent with you or something."

That was enough to start the floodgates. Finding a spot to sit, she gave me a handful of Kleenexes. But once the tears had started, they would not stop.

As I made an effort to stem the flow of tears, I asked her what the doctor had actually told Larry.

"He said that Larry could leave when he had some things in place like being able to use the crutches well on the stairs. You should ask the doctor what you can do about his behavior."

She came to the nurses' station with me and spoke to the doctor because I was still in a very upset state. "Is there some medication he can be taking to calm him down?" she asked.

"He's a very abrasive and difficult man," the doctor answered. Looking at me he asked, "Do you think he will take medication?"

I wasn't sure that he would. "Can we at least try?"

Extending her visit, she kept me company while I tried with difficulty to control my tears. After I had calmed down somewhat, our friend left and reluctantly I returned to his room. I had been dreading coming to the hospital that morning; it had been the longest drive I had made to date.

Back in his room Larry continued to be belligerent, nasty and difficult. At 4:00 p.m. I stood up. "Well, I can't see much point in staying here any longer. I'll see you tomorrow."

"Don't bother if you've got something better to do."

"Based on your attitude, I can think of a lot of other things I would rather be doing but I'll be here." I leaned over and gave him a kiss.

I had decided that because it no doubt was his brain injury that was making him behave this way, I would try to help him through it. But I was not going to continue to tolerate being treated as he had been treating me.

When I arrived at the hospital the following day, he was surprised to see me. They had given him the medication the night before but he was complaining about it making him drowsy. "I'm not going to take it if that's the way it makes me feel. I don't need to sleep twenty-five hours a day."

Shortly after I got there one of the nurses came into his room and plunked down his pill. "Here's your pill. I hear you refused it this morning."

"I'm not taking it. I don't want to feel so tired and drowsy."

A Roller Coaster Ride With Brain Injury (For Loved Ones)

"What about if we gave you half a dose until your body gets used to it? Will you try that?" He reluctantly agreed.

As I left for the day and gave Larry a kiss, he said, "I love you."

"You are definitely testing my love," I responded.

On my way out I passed the nurses' station and the same nurse called to me. "You have to take care of yourself," she warned me. Because I had been so close to tears for days, they again began to spill down my face. "You must make sure that you set boundaries," she told me as she gave me a hug.

The next day he again refused the pill and was quite nasty with the nurse. "I'm just trying to do my job," she told him with a shrug at me before leaving the room.

That was the beginning of his bad mood for the day. "When exactly is ICBC going to put in the railings?" he ranted.

"They said they will phone me when they're coming out but I haven't heard yet. They said they will do it to work around my schedule of visiting you."

He glared at me, then continued on another rant. "I want to get some phone numbers so I can start phoning clinics and get my therapy started."

"You don't have to do that. ICBC takes care of referring you to a clinic but you won't go until you can weight bear."

"Well I may as well just stay here if I can't weight bear." From there his conversation started going around in circles, not making much sense at all.

A friend who had been visiting him while he was in this argumentative and critical mood decided it was time to leave. I was wishing I could go with him. Leaning over Larry he said, "Be good to this girl. You've got a good woman here."

After the friend had left I said, "You know you're not making it very pleasant for me to come and visit you."

"Well then maybe you should just save yourself a whole lot of trouble and not bother coming in until it's time for me to go home."

Laughing I said, "You could have said that you would try and be civil to me." I waited for a response that I didn't get. "I don't think your treatment of me is fair Larry," I added.

He looked at me before speaking then shrugging said, "It probably isn't."

I further commented that he seemed to make an effort to treat his other visitors civilly and politely. Why," I asked, "instead of being nasty with me, can you not treat me as well as you treat some of them?"

He stared at me for a few minutes and finally said, "Well if you want, I can be nasty with them as well."

"That doesn't make sense."

He shrugged again and refused to talk.

Another nurse came in and spoke with him and convinced him to continue taking the pill.

An e-mail received from a relative of Larry's on November 5th:

'Thanks so much for keeping us constantly informed on Larry's progress. We think and talk of you often. What a terrible time you and Larry have had to go through so far. Set-backs are not easy.'

My response:

'Hello to both of you;

Yes, it has been very difficult although Larry is coming along amazingly well. He only has two and a half more weeks and he'll probably be able to weight bear. He is now using crutches. ICBC came and did a home assessment and they are coming this week to put in railings to help him get around in the house. It has been a roller coaster ride – some good days but lately some very bad days. He has been difficult to get along with recently –

A Roller Coaster Ride With Brain Injury (For Loved Ones)

whether it's his frustration at being in the hospital or entirely his brain injury, I don't know. The doctor has now given him a medication to make him less abrasive especially with the staff and myself. He seems to have lumped me in with the staff. I guess because I try to explain things to him and he thinks I'm backing the 'bad guys' (the doctors and nurses). The last two days have been considerably better though because of the medication and I do hope he will continue to use it.

He has been referred to the Acquired Brain Injury Program which will assist him in his brain injury recovery – if there are any deficits he doesn't recover, they will help assist him in how to adapt to his deficits. He is determined to get out of the hospital although the staff is wonderful. I have found them to be very approachable and they have listened to my concerns and have acted on them. When he does come home there is a place not far from us where he will do his therapy. If his bad moods can be controlled with medication, I'm sure all will be fine – it'll be a time of healing.'

Later, speaking with the ICBC therapist she asked how Larry was doing.

"He's being very difficult and cantankerous. He says he'll be better when he gets home."

She was silent for a minute. "They usually think things will be better when they get home but then they discover they have another whole set of challenges that they find just as frustrating and so they are just as difficult." Another pause, "But maybe he won't be."

    I'd been cutting my visits down from six or seven hours a day to two or three hours because there had been many days when it was very difficult to spend so many hours at the hospital visiting him when he was being so confrontational. I was beginning to dread him coming home from the hospital.

    The following day I reluctantly dragged my feet down the hall to his room. He was sitting on the side of his bed. "Surprise, surprise," he said with more than a hint of sarcasm in his voice. "I didn't expect to see you."

    Friends had asked us for dinner but he had previously adamantly refused to go. "T.... and G...... were in today and they said dinner is for N....'s birthday so I said I would go for dinner," he told me as if he was giving me the best present in the world.

    "I'm glad you are," I answered. "Have you been out walking around with your crutches today?"

    "No. They told me that I can't go out of the room unless a nurse is with me."

    Later asking at the nurses' station, they said that was not the case. One of the physiotherapists later came to his room and told him he was allowed to go out of his room whenever he wanted to use his crutches. He never did.

A Roller Coaster Ride With Brain Injury (For Loved Ones)

The Medical Suppliers called to say they would be putting the railings in that Thursday. I have to admit that my heart sank a little with that phone call because it would only be a short time before Larry would be home. 'Would I be able to handle it?' It is sad to say that I was dreading his homecoming just as I was coming to dread my visits to the hospital to see him. It was difficult to turn my feet in the direction of his room knowing that each day when I stepped over the threshold I was laying myself open to more criticism, complaints and nastiness. It was starting to wear on my nerves and tears were always near the surface, if not already cascading down my cheeks by the time I reached the hospital. On the drive there I often tried to divert my thoughts to things unrelated to Larry's accident in an attempt to hold my tears at bay. But as I pulled into the parking lot each day I could not deny our reality and the tears always fell. And when he saw them, it seemed to give him more ammunition for his nastiness.

Larry got an evening pass and we went to dinner at our friends' house. Before his friend dropped him off that evening I told him I wouldn't be in the next day because they were putting the railings in. A friend came over for a visit on that afternoon and we were able to enjoy a truly relaxing and enjoyable day; one of the few I'd had since the day Larry had his accident.

The interesting thing with Larry was that he was able to make the effort to be pleasant, cheerful and friendly when we were out for dinner, but he could not seem to make the same effort towards me when we were alone.

November 9th e-mail to a friend:

'Thanks again for the lovely dinner and very nice evening. And also thank you to T... for driving Larry back to the hospital. ICBC came and did the railings today and they brought crutches and a wheelchair for him as well. He is quite insistent that he doesn't need a wheelchair but the therapist said one should be available even if he just uses it a couple of times. She also said there will probably be a lot of improvement in the next three months because there's usually a lot in the first six months, with regards to brain injuries. She said they would then see what his requirements are after that. She also said if he's difficult they'll have a caregiver come and relieve me and lay down the rules to him. But we won't know what he's going to be like or going to need until he gets home. A friend came over this afternoon for a visit while the fellow was here doing the railings. We had a nice chat and a glass of wine.'

I felt that he no doubt would be expecting that he could go home on the Friday. I phoned the hospital to let them know about the railings and what I thought he would be expecting.

"He'll have to be discharged by all of the departments and the doctor isn't back until Monday so he probably won't be discharged until Monday or Tuesday."

I felt some relief; I had a reprieve for a few more days.

On the Friday the therapist came to talk to Larry since time was short until his release from the hospital. "Let's try the stairs again," he suggested. I watched, at the therapist's suggestion, so that I could see how he was supposed to properly do it. When we got back to the room he told Larry when his next x-ray appointment was going to be.

"Now remember Larry you have to keep your weight off that left leg. Your x-rays on the 29th of November will determine when you will be able to weight bear. You'll know when you have put too much weight on your leg because it will feel achy. Also, remember you won't be able to drive for a minimum of six months."

"I'll lose my business if I can't drive for that long."

"You've already been here for three months. If that was the case, you could have lost it in three months also. It is a standard practice for people with brain injuries. There will be a process for getting it back.

"Also," he continued, "it's very important that you don't drink for two years because alcohol inhibits the healing process of the brain."

"Two years?"

"Two years. Smoking also slows down the healing process of the brain because it restricts the blood vessels so there is less oxygen going to the brain."

Looking around, the physiotherapist attempting humor said, "Now what other bomb shells can I drop on you?" He smiled kindly. "You'll probably be able to go home either Monday or Tuesday."

Larry had a day pass on the Saturday for one of my son's birthday. For the most part it was a good evening and everyone was relaxed – some were watching the hockey game in the family room and others were chatting in the living room. About 8:00 p.m. Larry decided he wanted to go back to the hospital because his leg hurt and he was tired.

"Why don't you lie down on the couch Larry?" one of my daughters-in-law asked him.

"No," he said quite adamantly.

"Should we move the coffee table over so you can put your leg up on it?" another daughter-in-law asked.

"No. That won't help."

"Why don't we get some pillows to put under your leg?"

"No, I just need to lie down."

A Roller Coaster Ride With Brain Injury (For Loved Ones)

His daughter was taking him back but she wanted to see the end of the hockey game and I didn't feel I could go and leave everyone. As a result he spoke little to anyone until his daughter was ready to take him back at 9:30 p.m.

To a friend:

'We had the dinner on Saturday. His mood wasn't initially bad although he was very harsh with one of the grandchildren a few times. He used to be very patient with him. Later he became cranky and wanted to go back to the hospital because he said he was tired and his legs hurt. I suggested an aspirin but he said no. I was surprised that he was in such a hurry to get back to a place he hates so much and wants to get out of. He was also very quiet. He hardly said a word the entire evening. I was wondering if it was because he wasn't drinking. But he did agree to continue with the medication when he came home so that is a good thing.'

My brother phoned from Mexico the next morning and told me if I want to run away I can always house-sit at their place while they're away and then I can stay at their place in Mexico while they're here. I could be a gypsy, he said. The thought definitely had some appeal after the previous three months. The reality is that I would never be able to be away from my family and grandchildren. And also who would look after Larry?

On the Sunday some friends came to visit Larry. While they were there, one of his nurses came in, "Here's your 'make you nicer pill'," he smiled.

"Larry, have you been hard on the staff?" the friend queried.

"I have been cantankerous to some of the staff," he admitted.

"And me," I added, again feeling the sting of tears that were always so close to the surface.

"Hang in there," the friend said as she gave me a hug when they left and I felt those cursed tears well up again. And once started, they wouldn't stop.

The friendly cleaning lady came in and said, "Ah, my girlfriend is here." Then taking a quick look at my face she asked, "Are you alright?"

I nodded and she left immediately. A few minutes later the nurse came and asked if everything was alright. The staff had been very good.

The surprise was that when I went to leave that day Larry said, "Thank you. I love you."

"You don't act like it most of the time."

"I know I haven't been." And he did look upset.

* * * * * * * *

The friend who had been for a visit to the hospital called the next day saying, "You looked at your wit's end yesterday."

"I am just about. Larry has been so difficult and I am either crying or on the verge of tears all the time. I don't know if I can keep handling how he treats me."

"I've always thought you two were a perfect match for each other."

"We were," I sighed. "We almost never disagreed about anything. I just can't believe that everything could change so drastically. I just hope that he goes back to being the person he was because I have to admit that I don't much like who he is right now. He's not the person I said I would live with."

* * * * * * * * *

The doctor wanted to talk to me to see if I thought I could handle Larry before they would agree to discharge him. Larry knew the doctor wanted to talk to me and why. He also knew that what I said would have a bearing on when he would be allowed to go home. He admitted that even with the medication he would have to make an effort to overcome his bad behavior.

One thing I have always been fortunate with is that I do have a lot of support from family and friends. Being able to talk about the situation was helpful and good, but once I was back in the room and seeing and hearing how he treated me, the memory of the support very quickly would fly out the window. I would be back in the lion's den looking down the throat of the enemy – an enemy that never before was.

* * * * * * * * * *

For the next three days Larry behaved fairly well. He knew he had to.

"Why," I asked when things were going well, "do you argue so vehemently about everything and emphatically state that you are right and everyone else is wrong? No one is going to tell you something is when it isn't. If you realize you have a brain injury maybe, just maybe you might be the one who has seen the situation incorrectly."

"If I behave that way when I get home, you should take a stick to me."

"There have been times that have been pretty scary with how you have treated me, like when your eyes have bulged in anger and you've bared your teeth at me," I told him.

"I remember you told me never to look at you again like that. But I don't remember why. I will try to behave better."

On the Tuesday before Larry's discharge, I talked to the assistant occupational therapist and she told me they had been slowing down Larry's discharge because of his behavior and because of their concern about me and how he will be when he gets home.

I also talked to the doctor. "I think he'll be fine as long as he continues to take his medication; at least I hope he will be," I told him with as much confidence as I could find. My words were spoken with much more bravado than what I was actually feeling.

An e-mail sent to everyone on my list:

'Just to let you all know that Larry is getting out of the hospital on Wednesday, November 15th. He is now using crutches and has about three more weeks before he can probably weight bear on his left leg. He will have to go for x-rays on November 29th to confirm that he will be able to at that time.

Larry had a day pass on the 11th so that broke into the time he had left in the hospital. He is very upset that he can't drive for six months – apparently that is standard for people with brain injuries. He also is not supposed to drink for two years because alcohol inhibits the healing process of brain injuries. He appeared to take the 'not drinking' much better than he took the 'no driving' news. He still has a lot of challenges ahead of him but the worst is hopefully behind him.

If you wish to come and visit, just give us a call to confirm that we are home.'

An e-mail from one of the recipients of the above:

'Thanks for the news. We hope Larry will get through the coming months with as few challenges as possible. Once Larry is home my hope is that he will start improving more as he has time to focus on things other than a hospital room wall.'

CHAPTER TEN

The End Of The First Phase

November 15

Larry was leaving the hospital! He was happy to be going home and I was fearful of what I might be facing.

Before we left I talked to the social worker. She gave me information on the Acquired Brain Injury Program which Larry had been referred to. I went around and thanked his regular staff – they were wonderful to him even though he hadn't appreciated them and had treated them poorly.

To a friend:

'The doctor wanted to talk to me before he discharged Larry to get my assurance that I felt I would be able to handle him. I wasn't sure but felt if he continued with his medication that hopefully it would be alright.

I was talking to Larry and he said that he can see things very clearly in his head and even if someone says it isn't so, he won't believe it because he has seen what he believes so clearly. I tried to tell him that no one is going to tell him things that aren't true – we're not trying to confuse him. He also said that even with the medication, he has to make an effort to control his behavior.

A Roller Coaster Ride With Brain Injury (For Loved Ones)

We stopped at the neighborhood drugstore and filled Larry's medication prescriptions on the way home; a number one priority on my list. The rain pelted; the wind ripped branches from the trees and my hair whipped wildly across my face. Many of the stop lights were out; it was a truly miserable day.'

We weren't home two hours when our power went out so instead of the steak and potato dinner I had planned for Larry's homecoming, we sat down to a meal of peanut butter sandwiches. Sitting around the gas fireplace in the solarium, we watched the trees bend grotesquely while the winds roared around the corner of the house. To make matters worse it wasn't long before the rain found several places in the roof of the solarium to drip through. By bedtime we had seven containers catching the errant water. Our power was out for fourteen hours. To be optimistic, the roof only leaked in the solarium; we did have the gas fireplaces to keep us warm; we had lots of peanut butter and Larry's mood seemed to be fairly pleasant.

His pleasant mood continued to reign next day. The following morning I said, "I know you're putting weight on your leg but I'm not going to nag you about it. You know what the consequences are and you are the one who will have to live with them. But I AM going to insist that you take your medication because if you don't, I will be the one who has to bear the consequences of that. And I don't intend to." He took his pill.

Two days later the ICBC therapist came out and talked to Larry to see how his adjustment to coming home was going. "I'll make a referral to the physiotherapy clinic for you," she told him, "and then you can call and set up a convenient appointment for yourself. The first appointment will be an assessment."

"The best therapy I can have is coming home," Larry told her.

Over the next few days I found that he just sat and looked out the window and had no interest in doing anything. Unfortunately, he doesn't read and has very few interests. I made a few suggestions but he followed up on none and I was beginning to feel guilty when I did things on my own even though I was still in the house. And if I didn't talk, he didn't. I felt as if I should be constantly entertaining him. I was also beginning to get a very bad cold and cough and was not feeling very well.

On the weekend we went to one of the grandchildren's birthdays and Larry sat in a corner (as he had at the last family dinner) and was very subdued, not making any effort to participate in the conversation around him. He walked around the whole time, using neither his crutches nor a cane. That night he was up in the night with pains in his legs. I said nothing. He knows the consequences.

For the next few days his mood stayed fairly even, although he continued to be unmotivated to do anything. "I have a couple of ideas of things you could do if you want," I suggested.

"I can't do anything. I can't walk."

I said nothing while I watched him walk around listlessly with neither cane nor crutches.

* * * * * * * * * *

"I won't start you on anything too strenuous until we get the okay from your surgeon," the physiotherapist told Larry at his assessment. "You're very fortunate to have no damage to your tendons or ligaments. It's amazing considering how much damage was done in the accident. With no tendon or ligament damage, it will cut down on your recovery time considerably."

An e-mail sent to friends on November 20, 2006:

'Hello Everyone,

'We are planning to have our combination 'welcome to our new home' party and our annual 'pre-Xmas party' on December 9th. We look forward to seeing all of you to enjoy the beginning of Christmas celebrations.'

For the first couple of weeks it was fairly busy between looking after grandchildren, taking one to school, having a couple overnight, doing Xmas baking, helping two grandchildren do gingerbread houses and putting up Xmas decorations and Xmas trees - some with the help of grandchildren - and doing the things Larry required. I also had begun to do Xmas shopping.

An e-mail to a friend on November 23, 2006:

'Larry is doing much better than I thought. With his little 'magic pill', his mood is good although I can tell when it starts to wear off. If I'm a little late getting it to him he starts to get a little edgy. Otherwise I notice some things that from my research are consistent with brain injuries but are things that are not glaring and probably wouldn't be noticeable to others, i.e.: he'll sit and do nothing because he says he can't walk but he's walking; he's unmotivated; he'll tell people that he can't put weight on his leg and that he's using crutches around the house but he almost never does; he's self-centered and his reasoning on many things is off. He's quieter especially around others which either may be the brain injury, his medication or the fact that he's not drinking. But it is early days and there is a lot of time left for healing. He has improved so much already that I really don't think there will be too much that won't be recovered. He's very fortunate.'

During this time the house was very cold and we could not get the thermostat properly regulated. It was not a major problem until the weather turned extremely cold and we began to get worried about it. We called a heating company to come and investigate the problem and were told the furnace was not hooked up to the thermostat. In the cold snap and the huge snowfall we had been forced to

A Roller Coaster Ride With Brain Injury (For Loved Ones)

wear our coats inside the house; and when the problem was resolved the ice slowly began to melt from the inside of the upstairs windows.

Over the first two weeks I noticed Larry hadn't become nasty or irritable like he had been in the hospital. He was, however subdued and withdrawn, initiating no conversation. When we talked it only continued as long as I talked. He made no effort to continue with the conversation. With my cold, sore throat and difficulty speaking, I became aware of how quiet the house could be when I was unable to talk.

Another thing that became very obvious was that he made no effort to be affectionate with me and in fact had a very different attitude toward me than before his accident. He didn't appear to have any concern for my feelings. It was more like neighbor to neighbor although I thought he probably would have made more effort to be friendly with the neighbor. Did he still have the capacity to feel, I often wondered? The problem might have been that he viewed me as his caregiver instead of the equal relationship we once had, or perhaps he perceived that I was the one with the power and there may have been some resentment. I didn't know; I had many unanswered questions. We used to laugh often. There were no longer any laughs. He occasionally smiled but he didn't laugh.

I also realized that his values and his attitude on certain issues had changed quite drastically. I didn't know if he was who he might once have been but he was no longer who I thought he was. I didn't know; we had only known each other four years before his accident. He was definitely not the same person I thought I knew.

He often perceived things quite differently than what they actually were. When he looked at the x-rays he saw a mess of crooked screws. When I looked at the x-rays I saw a wonderful job of straight precision. He swore they were crooked and he would never hire 'that guy' as a carpenter.

I asked Larry at one point if he felt much different. "Yes," he answered, "but I can't say in what way. I feel awkward. No, that's not the proper word," he said. "I can't say what the difference is."

He appeared to be feeling very sorry for himself. That seemed to be his primary concern.

He also appeared to be completely unaware that his accident had been very difficult for me too. He showed little or no appreciation for anything I did or for the fact that I had tried to help him over the previous few months - by encouraging and doing the cognitive exercises with him, visiting him almost daily while he was in the hospital, and looking after him when he got home. I felt strongly that there may have been some resentment towards me for those very reasons.

An e-mail from a friend on December 4, 2006:

'I was just wondering if you are available for coffee tomorrow afternoon.'

My response:

'I would like to. Larry is almost like he was before he was taking the medication – not quite as bad but negative with a bad attitude and making no effort to do anything. I phoned the ICBC therapist and asked if it was possible for him to see a counselor. He probably won't agree though. She's coming on Wednesday afternoon.'

Then things began to change drastically.

CHAPTER ELEVEN

Not Taking It Personally

Around this time things began to get very bad again. "I know I'm an a--hole," he told me.

"If you know that, why wouldn't you make an effort not to be?" I asked him.

"I don't feel like making an effort to change," he answered.

"I don't like the way you treat me." I didn't know which was worse – the tears that were never far away or the constant feeling of nausea.

"I don't feel like making an effort to do anything. It isn't just you, it's everything. You just happen to be here."

I phoned the ICBC therapist after this exchange. "When things become difficult," she told me, "you may just have to get out of the house for a while."

I took her advice and went Xmas shopping. When I came back three hours later, I could see that he was even angrier than he had been before I left. I assumed the fact that I had left accentuated the reality that he was stuck in the house with no means of leaving.

"I'll have dinner ready in about twenty minutes," I told him.

"I'm not hungry," he answered angrily as he limped his way upstairs to bed. It was 6:00 p.m. and he didn't come down for the rest of the evening.

The following morning I came downstairs about fifteen minutes after him to see him sitting at the dining room table playing solitaire. I proceeded to make him a breakfast of scrambled eggs and toast. When I placed it in front of him he said, "I've already eaten."

Looking around I saw nothing to indicate that he had eaten. "You have to eat Larry. You didn't have dinner last night."

Baring his teeth and glaring at me he said, "If I want to eat, I'll eat. If I don't want to eat, I won't." He seemed to be going out of his way to treat me as badly as he possibly could – once again.

He gathered up his bills and I asked if he would like to go to the bank. "You can drop me off at the bank," he growled.

Looking at the snow and the ice on the sidewalks and he with his crutches, I said, "I'll wait for you. It's dangerous to walk in this stuff with your crutches."

"I'm not coming back and you can wait until you're blue in the face. I'm going someplace else," he scowled. It was hard to believe that a face could change as much as his had but the change was scarily dramatic.

"Where are you going? I'll drop you off there."

"Never mind where I'm going. I'll take a taxi."

I let him out of the car and, with not much alternative, I came home. I then e-mailed his daughter at work.

'Your dad is even worse today. Yesterday when he was behaving so badly I phoned the ICBC therapist and she said to go out. I did give him his pill although he wouldn't eat breakfast. He insisted I leave him at the bank. He said I could wait until I'm blue in the face. I asked him why he's behaving like this and he said it's going to get a lot worse before it gets better. He also said he didn't know why and he doesn't feel like making an effort to change his behavior. When I dropped him off he wanted the house key but I needed it to get back into the house. This made him even angrier. He said if I wasn't home when he got home he'd kick in the back door.'

I then called the ICBC therapist. I was very upset and worried that he would fall on the ice.

Both his daughter and the ICBC therapist phoned and were here in less than two hours. Angela went looking for him and found him wandering down a side street. When she brought him back he glared at me with intense anger and hatred on his face before he limped upstairs. We left him for about an hour and then she went up and talked to him.

When she came down she said that his biggest thing was that all of his independence had been taken away from him and I'm one of the ones who had taken it away and the one who was telling him what to do. Unfortunately, that is the role of a caregiver for one who can't rationalize and be aware of what could cause him harm. He was also angry by the fact that his license had been removed. He also told her that he wanted to get rid of this house and move into a condo and then go to Hawaii. He told her he was down the side street looking for a real estate office when she found him so he could get rid of the house. The side street is residential. I personally think he was looking for the pub because he was headed in that direction.

After Angela talked to him she convinced him to come down and have lunch which he ate and then he immediately went back upstairs again. He refused to acknowledge me when I put his lunch on the table. The therapist arrived a short time later. She gave us a more in-depth explanation of head injuries than I had so far heard before she went upstairs to talk to him.

After talking to him, she said she would organize a taxi account for him so he could go to the clinic and to his doctor appointments on his own so he would feel more independent. She also said I should back off on everything except if there was an issue of safety involved. (Walking around in the snow and ice with his crutches was a safety issue, I believed). He didn't like me helping him with things and in plain words he wanted me to 'butt out'. He wouldn't take his medication on his own, though so I was to continue to do that and the therapist said if he refused to take it they would send someone out so that I didn't have to get into an altercation with him. She said, "Don't take it personally."

Although that is what everyone says, it is very difficult not to take it personally when a person is looking directly at you with anger and hatred on their face. I do believe, if only at that moment, there is a personal nature to it. Larry was including me in with everyone else who had taken his independence away and I believe he hated me for it as much as he hated them.

She suggested that, although Larry probably wouldn't agree to speak with a counselor, she thought I should. I was beginning to think I would need to because I was really starting to feel the stress of the whole situation. And how I felt about him was definitely altering.

I phoned his doctor for an appointment for the following day, at the therapist's suggestion. She suspected depression and when I talked to the doctor he said he had suspected it the last time he had seen him. He said that depression is very common with people who have had brain injuries, especially when they have also had other multiple injuries. The therapist explained that it was a chemical imbalance in the brain. She said when the body is severely injured everything goes into the body to repair that damage and the brain is left with a chemical imbalance because the body considers that the brain isn't the most important thing. She said most people stay on the medication for about six months and the brain by that time is producing enough chemicals and the patient can gradually be weaned off their medication.

The ICBC therapist asked Larry if he wanted her to help us reconcile but he said, "No, we'll work it out."

I wasn't so sure. There had been a lot of hurts that were difficult not to take personally. I had made a commitment to myself to stay until his brain had recovered as much as it was going to. But would I want to stay after that? I didn't have an answer. Would the feelings I had for him before the accident return? I no longer knew what I felt and I didn't know what the end result was going to be.

That evening a friend called and knew by my voice that something was wrong. I was still having difficulty keeping my shaky emotions until control. When I told her she said, "I know it's the brain injury but it's not right for him to treat you like that. It's so hard to understand – you two were like lovers from Camelot. He always said you were the best thing that ever happened to him; you were the 'apple of his eye'. But," she added, "people always turn on those they love."

"It's hard for me not to feel angry," I confided to her, "because for the last almost four months it seems my whole life has been trying to do what is best for him and the result is that he keeps 'smacking me in the face' at every opportunity he gets."

An e-mail sent to my mother because I was so upset that I wasn't able to talk on the phone after the day's experience with Larry:

'I've calmed down now. After you phoned K..... called. She said M... is going to be upset when he hears about Larry's behavior. Even though I know he can't help it – it still hurts. Sometimes things can't be forgotten. A friend was going to come over for a visit – I think he may not have wanted to be here when she came and that may be why he wanted to be left at the bank. I don't know. Larry's going tomorrow to see the doctor. He admitted to Angela that he wasn't treating me very well. She asked him to treat me better. Larry says he knows he's being an a...... but that's what he feels like being. The ICBC therapist thinks he's depressed and said the doctor will probably prescribe an anti-depressant. She tried to impress upon Larry how important it will be to take the medication. I hope tomorrow is a better day because it was hell today.'

The following day after telling the wife of a friend of Larry's how things had been going, she said, "You definitely had brought a gentleness out in Larry that wasn't in him before he met you. It's the brain injury. Why don't you act as if his

A Roller Coaster Ride With Brain Injury (For Loved Ones)

behavior isn't bothering you – hum and go about doing what you would normally be doing," she suggested.

This friend works with victims of brain injury and when I told her about Larry's wishes to go to Mexico or Hawaii, she said, "Quite often people with brain injuries feel that by going to a different geographical location things will be better but they still have the same problems - its just that it's a different place and different people. My concern is that he will become violent with you."

"Verbally he has been awful and if looks could kill I would be dead right now but I'm not afraid of him hitting me. At least I don't think he would do that."

December 6

We went to Larry's doctor in the afternoon. He did not go very happily, feeling it wasn't necessary. He spoke not one word the whole way there. In the office he chose to sit in another area of the waiting room from where I sat. However, when he was called into the doctor's office I asked him if he wanted me to go along and he surprisingly agreed.

The doctor asked specific questions to ascertain whether he was depressed or not. He also asked if he had felt this way while he was in the hospital and he said he had. I had suspected that he was depressed as far back as Royal Columbian Hospital but when he was not put on medication, I thought perhaps I had been mistaken. (I was beginning to realize that I should have persisted. Had the problem been dealt with at that time, would he have been so difficult and nasty?) His doctor prescribed an anti-depressant medication and mentioned to Larry, "Depression places a lot of pressure on a relationship and puts a lot of stress on a partner." During our drive home Larry again didn't speak to me.

At home, while I was making us a cup of coffee, I began to think about what a ridiculous situation we had fallen into. He definitely wasn't going to suddenly start speaking so it was up to me. "Do you remember before your accident we always said that we would be able to work out any problems we had?" I asked him. "Why don't we try to work this problem out?"

He said nothing, ignoring the fact that I had spoken.

"Would you like a hug," I asked when I received no reply?

"No, it wouldn't do any good," he grumbled.

"It might make you feel better," I said.

"I doubt it."

Placing his cup of coffee on the table at his elbow, I leaned over and gave him a hug anyway and he responded with a hug that indicated how desperate he was feeling.

"That feels better, doesn't it?" I tried to smile.

"Yeah," he agreed unsmilingly. The dam had burst and he had spoken – if only a few words.

CHAPTER TWELVE

Two Steps Forward One Step Back

A short time later I gave Larry another hug in passing and his spirits slowly seemed to improve and he began to talk a little more. It was difficult for me to initiate the 'hugs' when he had been so nasty to me for so long and especially when I had been getting nothing back for any of my efforts. At this point it was a completely one-sided relationship.

Later that day, I smelled cigarette smoke on him and in the ensuite. "Are you smoking," I asked?

Looking me straight in the face he said, "No."

He must have picked up the cigarettes when I dropped him at his bank the day before because I hadn't smelled it previously. This was very upsetting because of how strongly I felt about living with someone who smoked.

It was very disappointing also that he would begin smoking again when first he had been told that, along with drinking, it was harmful to the healing process of his brain injury. Secondly, I felt he was not treating me with respect by lying when I asked if he was smoking and I was especially annoyed that he would smoke in the ensuite and bedroom knowing how I felt about it. I wouldn't have been so angry if he had chosen a less mutual area.

The ICBC therapist called to see how things were going and to ask what the doctor had said. "The doctor put him on an anti-depressant medication. He got some cigarettes though – probably when he went to the bank yesterday. Are there likely to be serious repercussions with regards to his brain injury with him smoking?"

"Smoking restricts the blood vessels getting oxygen to the brain so that the healing process of the brain will be much slower. But I think that based on his present state of mind it would be best to pick your battles."

I told her about the hug and how he was now talking a little. She seemed unimpressed with my miraculous hugs. "With brain injury, its two steps forward and one step back," she reminded me.

I had a conversation with one of my sons. "Smoking, they say, is more of an addiction than heroin is," he said. "Perhaps he's going through nicotine withdrawals. That might have had something to do with his mood too. He's had to give up everything – his license, drinking and smoking. That's probably why he feels as if everything has been taken away from him – all of that and his independence."

My wise son was no doubt right to some degree but I still felt that he should have treated me with more respect than he was doing and should have discontinued smoking in the bedroom/ensuite. I had to admit that the lying and sneaking bothered me almost as much, if not more, than the smoking.

An e-mail to my mother:

'This morning wasn't great. Larry didn't say anything to me for the entire morning. I mentioned about going to the doctor and he grunted that we both don't have to go if it's just for pills; he said I could go on my own. I told him his doctor wasn't going to talk to me when he's the patient so he reluctantly went. After our hugs that I told you about his spirits seemed to improve. And he took his medications without any problems and said, "I don't know why but I feel a little better." I hope he's in good spirits tomorrow. When he went to bed he gave me a kiss and said he loved me. He hasn't done that for a while. "I know I haven't been acting very well lately," he told me when he kissed me.

I'm still impressed with ICBC. They have been very supportive.'

Determined to keep life as normal as possible, I continued with plans for the annual Cookie Exchange and our annual Pre-Xmas party. Some thought I was crazy to go ahead with these plans considering what had been going on with Larry but I needed something to look forward to that was fun. I did, however decide to combine the Cookie Exchange with the Pre-Xmas Party instead of having two separate events.

A Roller Coaster Ride With Brain Injury (For Loved Ones)

An E-mail from a friend on December 7, 2006:

'We're looking forward to the party. Keep up the fight, Sylvia. Better times are ahead I think....you've earned them. Don't lose your positive outlook, nor your good nature - both are invaluable. And in the coming weeks, if you need a break for a day, call me and I will come over so you can get some respite.'

My response:

'I've actually thought that time spent with his friends (because he hasn't had many visitors lately) would be a good thing – maybe even to go out for lunch or something so that he doesn't feel so closed in. He makes no effort to phone anyone. His mood improved yesterday afternoon and this morning so far compared to the last week. They say two steps forward and one step back – sometimes it feels like it's the other way around. His anti-depressant medication should kick in pretty soon. See you on Saturday.'

At the suggestion of the ICBC therapist, I assigned a friend of Larry's to keep a watchful eye so he wouldn't drink any alcohol at our party. A couple of other friends jumped on the bandwagon to help with this also. It turned out to be one of our most successful parties.

An e-mail to a friend who wasn't able to make it to our party:

'G...... took on the job of making sure that Larry didn't drink at the party. It definitely wasn't going to be me. Larry was very tired. We didn't get to bed until 2:30 a.m. and he's used to going to bed about 7:00 p.m. He spent a lot of time standing so his legs were pretty sore too. You could tell by looking at him that he was totally exhausted but he was enjoying the evening. I thought it might be good if he got together occasionally with friends, without me, so he feels that he is doing something on his own – even though before his accident we did just about everything together. I think he now perceives things quite differently. I told you about him sneaking smokes. What a shame to start smoking when he's been off them for four months. It makes no sense whatsoever to me.'

Her response:

'Oh, not smoking again! That is quite a setback. How difficult all of this is for you to adjust to. It's too bad he's lying about it. I think you need to get away.'

My answer:

'I've told Larry that I'm going Xmas shopping twice this week and after Xmas I've found a writing group that meet three times a month that I'm going to join and I'm going to find a gym out here that I can go to because when I've gone before I always feel so renewed. Exercising is a great stress reliever. Although right now I am feeling fine. When he was behaving so badly, I felt like I was being dragged on the ground through a bumpy field. Brain injuries really are a roller coaster ride and the problem seems to be that you can't really count on the good periods lasting, I don't think; it seems that things can turn around again just as quickly.'

We were going in to the lead-up to our busy Christmas season and I hoped that Larry's mood would stay stable. I was leaving him for short periods of time to do Christmas shopping. After speaking to several of Larry's friends to see if they would spend some time with him, over the next couple of weeks, three people took him out for lunch. His mood, with the help of the medication, perked up noticeably.

As a result of this he agreed, with some ambivalence, to attend a concert and to go to the home of friends where people he didn't know would also be. There were several occasions during this time where we went out or had company. These were big steps for Larry. Friends had recently asked us to go to a restaurant with them two weeks previously and he had said, "Not yet; maybe after Christmas."

An e-mail to one of my sons:

'Larry's mood seems to be much better; he's talking and he even set up the lighted reindeer in the front yard with the help of Nick. I don't know if it's the two steps forward, one step back situation and we are in the two step forward stage or if the hugs made such a difference or if the medication is now working.'

Larry's mood continued to be stable as we neared Christmas. He was now initiating kisses and was even laughing on occasion. He was becoming more open – his face even had a different look to it – it appeared more human instead of the robot appearance he had been exhibiting. I was hoping the steps forward were going to continue.

The ICBC therapist called to see how things were going with Larry. "He's doing quite well," I told her, "and the party went very well. He didn't drink anything and he seemed to be okay with it. Uh, I know its two steps forward and one step back but do you think there will be any more steps back?"

Laughing she said, "I wish I had a crystal ball but I don't. Things will probably go along well for a while and then he'll probably get bored with the exercises or something."

"Also, his lack of independence may hit him again. It's difficult to know what bump will set him off but there are very likely going to be more bumps along the way."

That wasn't what I wanted to hear. "He will probably also go through a grieving process about not being able to do what he once was able to do," she continued.

"I'm going to try and get him interested in other things," I told her. "A friend of ours also has some ideas that Larry may be interested in doing. Maybe that will thwart the grieving process."

"Maybe," she answered doubtfully. "Usually they go through the grieving process before they're interested in looking at other things to do. We'll do what we can to help him through this process."

CHAPTER THIRTEEN

Life Goes On

December 19

An e-mail to Larry's daughter:

'The anti-depression medication must really be starting to work because I've noticed a huge change in your dad over the last two or three days. His spirits are definitely up and he's been laughing and feeling more social. We've done a few things socially in the last week. He has another doctor's appointment tomorrow. Next week he goes two days for three hours and after New Years he begins going three hours a day for five days a week for his physiotherapy. It does seem to make him feel more independent being able to take a taxi back and forth to the clinic.'

December 20

It was another very busy day. My mother had her pacemaker replaced yesterday. I had taken her to the hospital and waited until she went into surgery and then my brother picked her up and brought her back here. She stayed overnight with us (and for several days after). The following morning we had an appointment with Larry's doctor so I put things out for her before we left. I also was looking after my grandson for the morning and we took him along with us to the doctors.

Larry told the doctor he was feeling pretty good. "I don't know if it's the medication or one of our 'chats'," he laughed with a glance at me.

Dropping Reilly off at daycare we stopped to check on my mother before meeting for a late lunch with some friends. We came back and while dinner was cooking I ran over and picked up another grandson to help him with his homework. During all of this, Larry's mood remained cheerful.

My two grandsons stayed over the night of December 23rd because my daughter had to be at the hospital early for an MRI on the 24th as a result of the Grand Mal seizure she'd had about a month after Larry's accident. I spent the day cleaning and preparing for our Christmas Eve festivities for our dinner and gift opening that evening.

December 24

The whole family was with us for our special Christmas Eve; twenty of us for a sit-down dinner. The evening went very well with only a couple of times where Larry got cranky and spoke harshly, particularly with the children, but the moments passed quickly.

December 25

There was a smaller group for Christmas dinner because most of my family was going to their partner's families for dinner since they had all been here on Christmas Eve. Our group on Christmas Day consisted of one of my sons and his fiancé, my mother and Larry's daughter and grandson. Larry's youngest son had come over in the morning and stayed for lunch.

Larry enjoyed the quiet day and the visit with his daughter and grandson.

December 26

For me it was one of those 'let-down' days after the weeks of extreme busyness. There should be a gradual withdrawal from Christmas. If somebody else was having something we would've gone but I didn't feel, after everything that had been going on, that I wanted to host another event. Larry seemed to enjoy the quiet day.

An e-mail sent to family and friends on December 28, 2006:

'Hello Everyone, This is a New Years greeting to wish all our family and friends a very happy 2007 and to thank everyone for the support they extended to me when Larry was so badly injured and was in the hospital for such a long period of time. That support, friendship and love helped me through a very stressful time and meant an awful lot to both Larry and myself. We are looking forward to 2007 and to sharing many happy times with all of you.

To our family and friends, thanks and all the best, Larry and Sylvia."

A response from a friend:

A Roller Coaster Ride With Brain Injury (For Loved Ones)

'Happy New Year to you too. Let's hope for a MUCH better year for you two in 2007. It's hard to believe Christmas and New Years have come and gone already. Just took the tree down and the house always seems so empty. Let's hope we start getting flowers soon. Take care. I'm always happy to meet for lunch or coffee.'

My response:

'Nice to hear from you. We'll definitely get together soon. I plan to take some time for myself in the new year – go to the gym, join a writers' club and visit with friends.

We had 20 for a sit-down dinner on Christmas Eve. Christmas Day was a much smaller group. For New Years the whole family went to a restaurant for dinner. We've decided that it's going to be a tradition from now on.

Ah, the tree! I've been putting off the inevitable but I'd better get at it too. Yes, spring never comes too soon. We'll get together soon.'

Another e-mail from a friend:

'I talked to your mother recently. She said you've been so busy with Larry over the past few months but she does seem to be a little worried about you. I hope everything is okay with you Sylvia. Wishing you and Larry all the best for 2007. We have to get together. Take care.'

My response:

A Roller Coaster Ride With Brain Injury (For Loved Ones)

'I know mom worries about me – the whole family has been although now that Larry is behaving better, they are relaxing somewhat. There were some pretty awful times I admit where if I wasn't crying I was constantly on the verge. I've had unbelievable support from family and friends which has helped. And ICBC have been terrific. But he's now on some wonderful medication so things have improved. Talk to you soon.'

* * * * * * * * *

During this period of time, Larry quite often said things that were incorrect. He seemed to get something into his head and was convinced that it was the truth and, even when corrected, he insisted that he was right. As a result it often sounded as if he was lying and he often contradicted entirely what I had said. An example of this was when one day I mentioned that Larry still slept about three or four hours during each day. He argued and insisted he no longer slept during the day. I suspected that the problem was memory-related.

He also said to people that at the scene of the accident they told him that twenty years ago they would just have put him in a body bag because he wasn't breathing. The truth was, he wasn't even aware of who was at the scene of the accident.

Another story he liked to repeat during this time was that they had to pump up his chest and that's why he had marks on each side of his chest when, in fact, the marks were where the drainage tubes had been inserted for when they were draining his lungs. He did this type of 'changing the story to fit what he wanted to say' and at times his story was very far removed from what we actually did or what had actually happened.

I told him one day about when my father had been hit by a car and thrown fifty feet and he'd had to get eight bone surgeries where they took bone out of his hips and put them in his legs. As a result one leg was three inches shorter than the other. After that, Larry began to tell people one of his legs was three inches shorter than the other.

Larry's stories were definitely interesting twists on reality – his being different than what the facts presented. Although I knew they related to his brain injury, I wasn't sure in what way.

January 2, 2007

Larry began his physiotherapy program. He would be going three hours a day, five days a week. He was not very happy when he came home after his first session. It was harder than he had imagined it was going to be and his body was sore. He got electrical therapy on his knee; he used the bicycle and treadmill machine and other weight machines as well as doing exercises on his own. I hoped it was not going to be another 'bump' in the road.

After the next two days of sessions he was in a better frame of mind when he came home and I thought he actually might enjoy himself. He got into a few conversations with others in the program which was a good social outlet for him. I didn't know how much conversation he initiated other than to tell the therapist each day, "We've got to stop meeting like this".

Larry was still smoking in the bedroom/ensuite. I hesitated for some time mentioning it to him again in case it would affect his mood. I didn't want another episode. Finally, I decided to take the risk. I brought the subject up, reminding him of how I had felt about him smoking before I moved in with him. I also asked him if he remembered he had been told smoking wasn't good for the healing process of his brain.

Looking me straight in the face he again denied that he was smoking.

"I can smell smoke on you. And I smell it in the bedroom and the ensuite."

He still continued to deny it.

About an hour and a half after our discussion, I went upstairs and again smelled fresh cigarette smoke in the bedroom. Going back downstairs I said, "I don't want to start an argument but why did you smoke upstairs again after we just had our conversation?"

He swore he hadn't.

January 9

A Roller Coaster Ride With Brain Injury (For Loved Ones)

Larry hadn't been staying at the clinic as long as they would like him to because his legs were quite sore.

When the ICBC therapist came today, Larry told her that he can't visualize an area when he hears the address; he knows where he wants to go and knows how to get there but couldn't explain to anyone because he can't remember the names of streets.

"I suggested that he look at a map book and re-familiarize himself with the names of the streets in the areas he's likely to be going," I told her. She said this was a good idea.

We had also been playing crib and I was teaching him to play hearts (when I could convince him but he was reluctant to try new things). I believed strongly that it was important to try and keep his mind active.

An e-mail from the ICBC therapist:

'I wouldn't mind meeting with Larry alone so I can do some cognitive activities with him – he wouldn't have you to rely on for backup info and sometimes I get a clearer picture of functional ability when a person is alone. Then, if you're home near the end of our appointment, you can join us. Is that okay with you?'

January 24

My response to the ICBC therapist:

A Roller Coaster Ride With Brain Injury (For Loved Ones)

'I'm confirming your visit with Larry on Thursday. One thing I thought I would mention is that he is still taking no initiative in doing anything – he does do crosswords and plays solitaire but not much else. This would be fine but when we were out with friends he was saying how bored he was during the day because the exercises are only in the morning. When he was in the hospital he was in such a rush to get home so he could do so many things but now he doesn't feel like doing them. The friend bought him a car model kit because he said when he was a kid he used to enjoy doing them. He says he'll probably do it someday but has shown no great interest as of yet. There are a lot of things he could do so as not to be bored but he doesn't make any effort. He will do things if I get him going and do them with him but this isn't always possible. It would be nice if he could be motivated to do some things on his own. Do you have any ideas? I suggested that he make a list of possible things he could do to pick from when he's sitting feeling listless and bored and doesn't know what to do. He agreed but probably won't do it. I'm quite concerned about his lack of motivation.

As far as his mood goes though, he is doing fine – a few cranky periods, mostly with the grandchildren and sometimes with me. He's been agreeable at social functions and seems to enjoy them. He still seems to be having problems with his memory. The other evening when we had company he told some stories – neither of which was entirely true. He seems to focus onto something he's heard and then makes a story up around it sometimes transferring it to himself when it has originally been about someone else.

After the people had left I mentioned this to him – telling him the actual story and reminding him of how he had changed it. Any ideas would be appreciated."

Response to my e-mail:

'Thanks for the update – I appreciate hearing your comments and concerns. I will respond to some of the concerns you have raised after meeting with Larry tomorrow.'

January 25

As usual we had several busy days. We had one of my son's birthday dinners with the whole family in attendance. And on another day friends came over for a visit. My friend and I kept up a steady stream of chat but the conversation between Larry and his friend was fairly stilted. He still was having difficulty keeping a conversation going or initiating any of his own.

Before his accident when we had company, Larry would participate in the preparation. He was now making no effort to do so. If I asked him to assist me with something, he did so without appearing to mind; but made no effort to initiate any further help. But he was always glad when I sat down because then he said he didn't feel so guilty.

Larry was still making no effort to take the initiative to be responsible for taking his own medication. He had to be reminded every day.

He was, however, making a bit more of an effort to be affectionate. He occasionally hugged me and also was giving me a kiss when he went to bed. Larry still seemed to be mainly preoccupied with his own concerns. This is one of the symptoms of frontal lobe brain injury – to be self-centered. This was not the Larry I knew before his accident. Also, pre-accident we discussed the few problems we had, always saying that nothing would be a major problem that we couldn't talk out. He no longer wanted to or was able to discuss problems. Possibly it was, as the ICBC therapist suggested, the fact that he was taking the medication and it was making his emotions very flat. Or it might simply have been lack of empathy which is also a brain injury symptom where a patient is unable to understand another person's feelings.

He was still finding it necessary to go to bed early; usually about 7:30 p.m. and he still seemed to require lengthy naps during the day.

January 31

Larry said he was beginning to feel a difference in his legs; he said he could see some progress.

Another thing that is different with Larry than it was before the accident is that his anger is more easily set off. Before his accident, he was very easy going and it took a lot to make him angry; in fact, I had never seen him really angry. Now I was becoming very afraid to tread in areas where I thought his anger may be inflamed. He tended to have a shorter fuse particularly where the grandchildren were concerned and quite often with myself.

An e-mail to a friend on February 11, 2007:

'We have been very busy this past week. We had to go to the Royal Columbian Hospital – a follow-up with the orthopedic surgeon – everything is fine; and we've had various visits with friends and family. Larry had his weekly meeting with the ICBC therapist and of course his daily physiotherapy. He also, along with Mike, lettered a truck one day and on another day they did a site-check on two jobs. Larry can't do either one but that's okay because they are thinking of doing other things. He also did one of those big checks for a charity organization. His spirits are improving and he's been staying up a little bit later at night too. We're going out with friends for dinner tonight.'

The e-mail response:

'It's all good news and the best news of all is your tone – it's optimistic and happy. Good for you. You will have to record this success (you and Larry have survived the worst and are moving on to more good things).'

A Roller Coaster Ride With Brain Injury (For Loved Ones)

An e-mail to another friend on February 13, 2007:

'There seems to have been a bit of a jump in improvement mentally with Larry with his attitude which is so nice. There has been steady improvement since Christmas. I mentioned holidays again to him and he asked where I was thinking of going. I suggested that we get our passports ready so we at least had them when we do decide to go someplace.

It's been almost six months since the accident. They told him he will be finished with his physiotherapy in about a month. He goes in April to the neurophyschologist for several appointments. The first one is for three hours. These apparently will determine when he'll be able to get his license back and where his weaknesses and strengths are. He's looking forward to doing the garage and some things in the yard but he's got it in his head that he can't begin until the appointments are over. I'm glad that he's beginning to be interested in things. He doesn't sound as if he's mourning the loss of his job yet. The ICBC therapist said that usually happens.'

Larry suggested taking me out for Valentine's dinner. I was impressed that he remembered and that he offered and that he did it.

And an e-mail from another friend:

'Larry, so glad to hear that you are doing so well! I have always known that you are a survivor.

A Roller Coaster Ride With Brain Injury (For Loved Ones)

As far as short term memory is concerned, I think I hear the buzzer on my stove telling me my water is boiling for coffee.

Keep up the good work. I'm sure the warmer weather will make those bones feel so much better. Thank you Sylvia for keeping us informed.'

An e-mail to all:

'Just to let everyone know that Larry has been told he will be finished with his physiotherapy at the end of March. He has noticed an improvement lately with his legs in that he can walk more easily and go up the stairs a little better and although they are painful during the week when he's doing his three hours per day five days a week regime, on the weekends they seem to be much better. They test him every few weeks and he is getting stronger and can do more each time. We haven't heard what Larry has to do to get his license back. He seems to have adjusted to and accepted the fact that he isn't going to be going back to doing what he once did – work-wise but he has some other ideas. The ICBC therapist comes once a week to work with him to improve his short term memory capabilities. On the 22nd, it was six months since his accident. Mentally, I think he has done amazingly well in that time and there is apparently a two year window for improvement with brain injuries. Our best to everyone.'

An e-mail sent to the ICBC therapist on February 25, 2007:

A Roller Coaster Ride With Brain Injury (For Loved Ones)

'I had mentioned to you before Christmas when Larry went through that bad period that he was sneaking cigarettes. You suggested at that time, considering his mood, that it wasn't the best time to mention it. I haven't until recently but felt forced to because he has been continuing to smoke in the bedroom/ensuite and I really do not wish to breathe in the smoke any longer. I also mentioned previously to you that he tells stories which amount to lies – a story built on a bit of fact. Is this insistence on doing what he wants regardless of anyone else a symptom of his brain injury? I'm very concerned about this lying. He is still a long way from being the person he was before the accident.'

Her response:

'I do not know where Larry's brain damage occurred as I do not have any medical records from his stay at Royal Columbian Hospital or Queen's Park Care Centre, however, his behavior could be related to the injury. Lack of insight, disinhibition, lack of self awareness and self monitoring, poor memory, impulsivity – all of these are behaviors that can be related to brain injury. Do you want me to discuss this smoking issue with Larry – if so I have to be able to say we have spoken?'

And my response:

'It was his frontal lobe area but exactly what portion of it, I'm not sure. I have no problem with the smoking issue being discussed with Larry and I don't mind that he knows I told you about it. I wouldn't mind though being there, or in the vicinity at least when you do bring it up in case he lies about it. It's the lying that is especially making me very annoyed. His problem shouldn't have to be my problem as well. All the way along I've been very clear about how I've felt about smoking. I haven't changed the rules. The behaviors you have mentioned – are there ways they can be dealt with? When I say he is not the same person; one way he shows this is when we talk. If I say something that would require a personal response with some emotion being the logical response, he has none. Thanks.'

February 25

    I went over to a friend's place to have a 'ladies only' evening and had a great time. I did feel guilty about leaving Larry alone for the evening but he seemed to be alright with it. He's usually in bed between 7:30 – 8:00 p.m. anyway.

February 28

    When the ICBC therapist brought up the issue of smoking with Larry, he said he knew I didn't want him to smoke upstairs and he remembered that I said I wouldn't move in with him because he smoked and he didn't know why he did it. I said if he wants to smoke, it's entirely up to him what he does with his body – all I'm asking is that he smoke somewhere else. I sensed he didn't get the point I was trying to make but he didn't seem to be upset with the fact that I had brought in the 'big guns'.

A Roller Coaster Ride With Brain Injury (For Loved Ones)

March 1

An e-mail from the ICBC therapist after my e-mail relating my concerns and her subsequent meeting with Larry:

'Following my meeting with you and Larry yesterday, I am of the impression that the emotional issue is mostly related to the medications, so you may see a change in him once he comes off the meds. The brain injury can cause an imbalance of brain chemicals that make it difficult to modulate mood and control emotions – you get the highs and lows, frustrations, etc. that you saw in Larry previously. Between the medications, exercise and time, it is hoped that the chemical balance of the brain will stabilize. His doctor will monitor that issue over time.

As for the other discussion about smoking, I am not certain that Larry could grasp what we were trying to say – that you didn't want him to smoke in the house. He seemed to interpret our discussion as that he should not smoke at all. It could be lack of insight, rigid thinking, impulsivity, lack of ability to self monitor, etc. that creates the situation where he smokes in the home, despite the fact that he knows you do not want him to. In any event, it seems to be related to the brain injury – he cannot see the problem for what it is and cannot self regulate to abide by the rules you both agreed to prior to the accident.

That doesn't mean that you don't continue to ask him to respect the rules, just that he may have

A Roller Coaster Ride With Brain Injury (For Loved Ones)

difficulty doing so. I hope that helps you in some way.'

My response:

'Thanks for the follow-up. I can understand with regards to the medication and agree that this will no doubt improve.

With regards to the smoking issue, which, as I said relates more to the issues of lying, sneaking and lack of respect, I later was convinced myself that it is his brain injury as well. In other situations he has done similar things, i.e.: when he wasn't supposed to weight bear, he continually told people that if he does he could end up back in the hospital for fifteen more weeks but he still continued to do it. The knowledge and the doing don't seem to have any connection. There have been other situations where what he says doesn't coincide with what he does – he just doesn't seem to get it sometimes. He seems to focus on something and he's like a dog with a bone on that one little thing like the fact that he couldn't smoke rather than the fact that the issue is to not smoke upstairs. Is it similar as with children, if they hear something 25 times in a row they get it – if I say it often enough, will he understand?'

And her response:

'You've made some good connections between similar circumstances and they appear to support the premise that Larry's behavior is related to the injury and not just him being disrespectful of you. Perseveration ('focus on something and he's like a dog with a bone on that one little thing') is also a common symptom of frontal lobe damage. I hate to categorize people's injuries, but these behaviors are indicative of a frontal lobe injury. Time will only tell whether Larry will improve in these areas. So, I don't know if you will have to tell him 25 times or 125 times, but I encourage you to discuss these issues with him as long as you have the patience to do so.'

Shortly after each discussion, Larry would go upstairs and have a smoke. He never quite seemed to get the concept of 'not smoking upstairs'. Each time when I mentioned it yet again, he would stare at me as if this was something completely new to him. If I said, 'we just had this conversation', he would shrug. He never knew why he did it. I began to wonder if what I thought we had before his accident had been an illusion. Were these tendencies there before and I hadn't known or had the brain injury really changed him so drastically? It is, I realize as I write this now, perseveration, another brain injury symptom.

Larry continued to operate on a 'he' level, not a 'we' level. I have discovered that until brain injury deficits can be adapted to, this is typical.

The ICBC therapist tried to encourage Larry to do Sudoku but he wasn't interested. Nor was he interested in 'word search' exercises (some of which I had already got for him) or some of the games they played. His interests are extremely limited which makes it difficult.

A Roller Coaster Ride With Brain Injury (For Loved Ones)

Larry still had cranky episodes, often relating to the younger children but also if I disagreed with him. At those times, he would become so angry with me that unless I felt strongly about something, I decided to avoid a discussion rather than disagree with him. I had never felt nervous before with him but when I'd see anger on his face when I disagreed, it was sometimes scary. It seemed to happen particularly when he got 'stuck' on an 'idea'. He couldn't seem to move beyond what he was 'stuck' on even when the 'real' story or the logical answer was pointed out to him.

March 10

We went to the home of friends for dinner. Larry started to make stories up. At one point he said that the lane he had turned into when he had his motorcycle accident was closed and there were red cones in it and he had no idea why he went into that lane. I said it hadn't been closed and there were no red cones. He yelled at me and became very angry. He said 'someone' had told us but he couldn't remember who the 'someone' was. I was told by both the ICBC adjuster and the RCMP lady that there was no signage, only a flashing light and a triangle on the mower. He became angry when I said that too.

The following day I asked Larry if he had anything to say to me for the way he had spoken to me. He said no. I asked if he felt I was due an apology for the fact that he had yelled at me, especially in front of people. He said no. I asked him, as I did another time, if he remembered what our relationship used to be like before the accident. He said, "Yes, it was wonderful." "How was it wonderful?" I asked. He didn't remember how, only that it had been. I told him some of the ways that it had been and reminded him that we had not talked like this to each other before; we had not yelled at each other and this was not how our relationship had been. He sat stony-faced. He was so angry he said he was going to put a 'for sale' sign up in front of the house. He was like a rock stuck in the middle of a path impeding the progress of everyone but so deeply entrenched it couldn't be budged.

Then I thought that perhaps he's been so cranky and difficult lately because his physiotherapy was coming to an end and he might be feeling a little unsure because of the change. He was thinking of his therapy as his 'job' and once that was finished, he'd be jobless.

I e-mailed the ICBC therapist my theory so perhaps she could address it with him when she came the next time. Then I gave him a hug and he calmed down and started behaving better. I suspected that, as a caregiver, it really was a one-way street.

The ICBC therapist had arranged for a kineseologist to work with Larry to help him with muscle control and possibly to go to the driving range with him. The commitment of having to spend time with the kineseologist is important because he wouldn't motivate himself to do things on his own otherwise. And I'm sure if I tried to get him to go to the gym on a regular basis and he didn't feel like it, there would be an argument.

March 29

Larry's mood was gradually improving and we did get along fine as long as I didn't disagree with him; I ignored his smoking and didn't try to 'un-stick' him from stories and ideas he was 'stuck' on.

He had appointments with an audiologist – his hearing I suspected, had been affected by the accident. The audiologist said that as the sounds became higher pitched, his hearing diminished. He also had his two front teeth repaired that were chipped in the accident.

The therapist was trying to get him to be responsible for taking his own medications – that had been a slow process. He depended on me to remind him. He was becoming a little more motivated to do some things – he raked some leaves in the yard and began work on his model car but still spent most of his time playing solitaire, doing crossword puzzles or sitting on the couch. He said his legs were still very painful. I wondered if they would be so painful if he got regular exercise and increased what he did each day.

His doctor said that's what he should be doing but when I suggested walks, he usually said his legs were too sore.

April 4

Larry had recently been doing more – we'd gone for a few walks; to the gym; he had gathered up the garbage for spring clean-up (and was taking the garbage out on garbage pick-up day – I had been doing that previously) and he occasionally took his dishes off the table and put dressings, etc. in the fridge; sometimes he would make us a Sunday morning breakfast and occasionally he made the bed. He was now totally responsible for taking his own medication although I always checked and still occasionally had to remind him.

April 11

Between friends and family the Easter weekend was very social. The following week we were looking after one of my grandsons and on the way, Larry insisted I had gone by the street we were supposed to turn at (I knew I hadn't, but decided not to argue).

I backed up and went the way he wanted me to go. We drove in silence for some time until finally he said, "I don't know how we missed Boundary."

"Possibly because we took the wrong turn," I suggested. He made no comment. I phoned my son to see how to get to his place from where we were. Nothing was mentioned by either of us but I felt that by letting him find out for himself that he was wrong, rather than disagree and have him get angry, was worth the extra miles it took to get to my son's place.   It was kind of a logical consequence exercise. Would he ever be who he once was, I kept asking myself?

The following day Larry had his first appointment with the neuropsychologist. We both met with him and he asked each of us questions to determine the background. Much of it Larry was unable to remember. Then I went out to the waiting room and Larry worked on exercises and was tested for over two hours; he thought they were problem-solving questions. He said he became frustrated with some of them because they were timed so he refused to do them.

April 16

We went to a second appointment with the neuropsychologist on this date and he had more tests – for two hours – he said they were mainly memory exercises. Larry was becoming a little more affectionate with me and seemed to be making a little bit more of an effort. I also hadn't smelled cigarette smoke for more than a week (he'd probably run out of cigarettes and hadn't found a way to get them again).

May 9

Larry had his last appointment with the neuropsychologist. Besides us, the ICBC coordinator and the ICBC therapist attended the meeting. He felt Larry had done fairly well in his testing. He also felt Larry was doing better at this stage of his recovery than other patients with similar brain injuries that he had dealt with and he

A Roller Coaster Ride With Brain Injury (For Loved Ones)

felt there was no reason why Larry shouldn't be able to get his driver's license back. He also suggested that it would be advantageous for Larry to see a counselor or a psychologist. The neurologist said he had noticed during the testing that Larry was easily frustrated and his irritability level was high. The ICBC coordinator said she would look into setting up a Driving Assessment for him to begin the process to get his license back and set up an appointment with a counselor. Larry cleaned the back pond and cut the back grass today. He seemed much more willing to do something; perhaps the good news motivated him.

His mood seemed to be much improved.

We also looked at a 28 foot motorhome which we were considering buying. I planned to drive it until Larry got his license back.

CHAPTER FOURTEEN

Bumps In The Road

May 21

Larry was back to being argumentative, nasty, disagreeable, cantankerous, belligerent, self-centered and downright unpleasant. He also again became unmotivated. If I didn't agree with him about something; he became very angry. He wouldn't discuss anything. He was very upset that he hadn't heard anything about the date for his Driving Assessment – that is what had set him off. It was another 'bump'. I e-mailed the ICBC therapist to let her know that he'd become very anxious about not hearing of a date for when he will be having the Assessment. She responded that she had heard nothing either.

May 22

On this date Larry decided that he was going to get the insurance on his own car because he was determined he was going to drive. I told him if he was going to drive when he didn't have his driver's license that I wasn't going to take him to get the insurance. He said he'd walk there. (Its about ten blocks each way). I told him I was going to let the ICBC therapist know what he was planning to do because he wasn't thinking properly and the way he was behaving indicated to me that he still had severe problems with his brain injury. He said he didn't care. He walked there and back to get the insurance for his car. (It was rather interesting that he made no comment about his legs hurting in spite of the long walk.)

June 9

Larry still had not got a date for his Assessment and was becoming angrier and more frustrated with each passing day. The I.C.B.C. therapist came to visit him and said, "I hear you've been getting a little bit cranky, Larry." She explained that things take time and he wasn't the only one waiting. She said that's bureaucracy. Larry had earlier angrily called the ICBC coordinator and said he was going to drive the motorhome to Kelowna on the first of July whether he had his license back or not. She told him she would make sure there were roadblocks up if he did. (I began wondering if they had slowed the process for him obtaining his license because of his high frustration and high irritability level as they did when they kept him in the hospital longer because of his poor behavior). I suggested to Larry that perhaps this was the case. I also suggested that perhaps they were not the ones to be having temper tantrums with because they were the ones who hold the power and determine when things are going to happen. He just became angrier with me.

During this period of time Larry continued to be very difficult. He was unable to contain his anger and frustration and took it out on me and the young grandchildren particularly. He seemed to be able to make an effort for other adults though. He also still continued to smoke upstairs. I gave up saying anything. It did no good and only made him more difficult. I tried talking to him in an effort to get him to attempt to contain his anger and frustrations but he always insisted that no fault lay with him, insisting instead that his problems were me, ICBC, the doctor or somebody else. Never himself. Larry kept insisting that he didn't need an Assessment to get his license back – he knew how to use a clutch and a brake. I tried to explain that it was a cognitive test as well as a physical assessment. He insisted that if it took much longer, he'd drive anyway.

August 13

In the past two months we got the bad news that my mother had breast cancer. She had surgery on July 12th and had her breast and lymph nodes removed. She stayed with us after her surgery. Two weeks after that one of my sons got married. It was a beautiful wedding and my mother was able to walk down the aisle on the arm of my eldest son.

Larry went through many emotions during the month of August. At times he was difficult and had many angry periods. A lot of his anger continued to be directed at me and several times I wondered if he was taking his medication. I continued to remind him about his medication because there were still times when he forgot. But there were occasional good periods too. The Assessment was finally set for August 15th. He still was not particularly motivated to do anything. If I suggested something, if he was inclined, he would do it, if not, he wouldn't.

We went away in our motorhome for the July long weekend with two other couples (I drove) and we had a very nice time. I was glad that the other couples were along because Larry had become very frustrated with the instructions for various things to do with the motorhome. He said the instructions may as well have been written in Japanese because he could not comprehend them. The two fellows very discreetly helped him. Larry was the same with directions when we traveled in an unfamiliar area – he became easily overwhelmed, sometimes throwing the written instructions at me. He did come out of his doldrums somewhat after that trip.

Once a date had been set for his Assessment, there was a very definite improvement in his attitude. Larry laughed more and was a little more affectionate with me. He became interested in working in the carport; closing it in to make a workshop and building a work table and easel. I suggested that he get a table saw. When he was busy and interested in something, he didn't complain as much about the pain in his legs; he noticed it more when he was sitting and doing nothing. He was also looking forward to us going away in the motorhome in September and possibly October if the weather was decent.

August 15

Larry had his Driving Assessment today. We arrived about 9:00 a.m. and he was given some cognitive testing; his eyesight was tested and they put him in a simulator to determine his responses before they took him out for a two hour road test. I was in with him for everything except the road test. As a result of his road test, they suggested that he take two- two hour driving lessons. He wasn't as upset as I had expected he would be but he later said he hadn't expected to pass anyway. It was a seven hour day between the drive in and back, the testing and the wait while he did his road test.

Later in the evening I asked him if he would come with me the next day to pick up my mother's dog at the veterinary after the dog's surgery. We had to take him to the after surgery care kennel and I wasn't able to lift him because I had hurt my back.

"Why can't the vet do it? he asked.

"Because that's not his job and also because he has MS," I told him.

"But then I'd have to wait while you go to the chiropractor," he complained.

I was fairly upset with his attitude and lack of willingness to help me in spite of the fact that I had spent so much time taking him to his Assessment and waiting for him.

He told me I shouldn't be so sensitive.

"Don't make me out to be the bad guy," I said. "I can't believe how selfish and self-centered you are." I felt bad the minute the words were out of my mouth but by then it was too late to drag them back.

"That's right," he replied angrily, "I'm the bad guy." He thumped his way upstairs to bed at 7:30. I tried to remember that he does have a brain injury but *'when will my feelings be considered'*? I asked myself. I went and got the dog by myself.

August 20

I took Larry to see the orthopedic surgeon on this date. Larry had been hoping that he would be able to get all the steel out of his leg. He had insisted all along that the doctor said he takes the steel out of 94% of his patients. I had not heard this, although I had been with Larry each time he had met with the doctor. When we met with the doctor he told Larry that, after looking at the x-rays, he could see that he was healing very well, especially considering the injuries he had sustained. When Larry mentioned taking the steel out, the doctor said it would make his leg weaker. He said it would be like putting a bunch of holes in a pipe – the pipe would be more likely to break. He tried to get Larry to pinpoint exactly where his pain was but Larry wasn't able to do so. He did say though that the left knee was the most painful. The doctor seemed to be reluctant to take the screws out but finally said that he may consider doing his left knee but he wanted to see him again in December to see how he was doing.

September 1

On August 25, 2007 my family (daughter and family), three sons and their spouses, and three grandchildren, as well as my mother came over with us to Gabriola Island. We always stay at the same place; we eat together and play games together. Larry interacted very little – most of the time he kept himself very separate from the rest of the family. He also wouldn't play games although in past years he has been part of the evening fun. But what particularly bothered me was his treatment of, and the way he talked to my four year old grandson. (Reilly's mother had gone back earlier). I spent most of the week trying to keep the child out of Larry's way. At one point, it was so bad I was tempted to return home but it would have ruined the rest of the family's holidays. I suspect that Larry was not in his comfort zone while we were over at Gabriola Island; perhaps he felt overwhelmed with so many people around in an area that wasn't his home. Whatever the reason, I have discovered that anything out of the norm tends to throw Larry for a loop. He is not good with changes or with anything that he perceives as a 'bump in the road' from what he's comfortable with.

September 11

I met two friends for lunch. They asked how things were going with Larry. I confided that I didn't feel appreciated – that he took everything for granted and that his behavior was still poor. Everything seemed to be an expectation and he didn't seem to feel that a 'thank you' was ever in order. I told them that I could hardly wait until he got his license so that he could be more independent. I was hoping also that when he got his license there would be a turnaround in his behavior and attitude. I was at a low point between Larry's behavior and my mother's illness.

September 13

We discovered that the cancer did not go into my mother's bones. We were all very relieved.

Larry had two driving lessons and on this date he went for his driving test and happily passed the examination. By this time between Larry's behavior and my mother's illness I said I really needed a break where I didn't have to do anything. I wanted to go away in the motorhome for a while and just relax. I said if he didn't want to go, I would go with a friend.

We decided that we would leave on September 16th for a week and drive a little and camp a little. I was looking forward to it.

September 23

We had a wonderful week in our motorhome; the weather was decent and it was very relaxing. I did only what I wanted and absolutely needed to do. Larry made no demands on me and seemed to be quite happy. He drove most of the trip and I think he enjoyed his new independence. There were no 'bumps in the road'.

CHAPTER FIFTEEN

Adaptations and Adjustments

Initially, I believed that as a person with brain injury improved, they would begin to learn skills to be able to adapt to and deal with any deficits they were left with. The ICBC therapist said that because Larry would not admit to her that he had any deficits, she was unable to help him any further and she closed his file. He did admit to me late in September, however, that he thought some things in his head would never be the same, although when I asked him, he had no idea what those deficits were. The ICBC therapist said many patients with brain injuries remain in denial their whole lives. I think for the most part Larry is in denial regarding the fact that he has any deficits.

Because his file had been closed, I did research on Internet to discover ways to help him adapt to his deficits. One study said, "Those with brain injuries must find different ways to deal with their new limitations. With help and patience, as well as using strategies and tools to compensate, they can often overcome their deficits. It also said that 'brain injuries can accelerate the decline of cognitive functioning as a person ages'. (Comments made by Lois M. Collins, Deseret Morning News). After reading this excerpt to Larry, I asked him if he was interested in trying, with my help to adapt to his deficits. He said, "Probably not."

His decision, I realized, left me with the challenge of learning to adapt and adjust to his brain injury myself, without his help. I decided, after thinking about the challenge, that adapting and adjusting was more a matter of coping and accepting.

According to McCubbin and McCubbin, 1991, the necessary requirements involve several important issues. First, there must be resiliency for there to be the ability to adapt and adjust to living with a family member with brain injury. Other important requirements included the following:

Personal Resources: They state there must be a) a sense of humor, b) physical and emotional health, and c) and a belief that one has some control over the circumstances of one's life.

Family Resources: For a successful adaptation to head injury there must be cohesion and adaptability in the family's capabilities to meet obstacles and shift courses. Families should also make an effort to maintain basic family routines and to create some degree of family continuity and stability. It is also important for families to have organization. These families have a higher probability of enduring. Also, on the Brain Injury Association's website it states that: 'active involvement of family and friends through the rehabilitation process is a key component to achieving maximum success.'

Social Support: Friends and the community are important as is how a family perceives an injured member's emotional and behavioral functioning.

A Roller Coaster Ride With Brain Injury (For Loved Ones)

Coping patterns include: 1) action taken to eliminate or reduce the demands created by the head injury, 2) acquiring additional resources not available to the family unit, 3) managing tension (both emotional and financial), 4) coping to make the head injury manageable and acceptable. Coping strategies play a critical role in adaptation. A family must work together as a unit through interdependence and mutuality.

There are many challenges associated with adapting to brain injury surrounding the injury; the long-term outcome, increased emotional and marital stresses, and the suppression of anger can present problems according to McCubbin and McCubbin, 1991.

Caregiving a patient with brain injury can present challenges relating to role changes, loss of sexual intimacy, empathetic communication and fewer social opportunities. It is important for families, states McCubbin and McCubbin to establish coping patterns rather than only adjust to head injury. There should be a sense of family control over environmental influences. Families will need to make changes in their priorities and goals.

Studies have found that as long as ten years post-injury there may be poor adaptation and adjustment to living with a member of the family with brain injury. In most cases, the deficits and differences in the individual are noticeable only to those who live with the affected individual. To others, they may seem fine.

EPILOGUE

Although Larry has done well and most people meeting him would likely be unaware that he had suffered a brain injury to the degree he did, those who know him well realize he is not the same person he was before his accident.

Our relationship is not the same as it was before his accident either. We do not talk as we once did, although conversation is slowly becoming a little more like the back-and-forth chat we once enjoyed. He still rarely initiates a conversation any deeper than occasional remarks, although I do see this very gradually improving over time. When we disagree on something, where before it was a discussion and debate, it now becomes frustration and anger on his part. Previously, he was very easy going. I didn't used to feel as if it was necessary to choose my words carefully for fear of angering him as I now do. While trying not to disagree, I will often be vague in my answers in potentially argumentative situations. I do however, see gradual improvements taking place as time goes on and I suspect that as long as there are no emotional setbacks, or bumps in the road, this will continue to happen.

Where before his accident he showed me in many ways that he cared and behaved in such a way that others also knew how he felt about me, this has been a very slow process forward. As time goes on, I believe there will be improvements in this area also and to a degree there already have been small steps taken. When he is no longer taking his anti-depressant and anxiety medication, perhaps he will be more emotionally like his old self. His doctor began the weaning process from both of these medications but when I realized that his frustration and crankiness became accelerated and his lack of motivation increased, I asked him to continue with his medication. By going back to the original dosage, Larry's attitude and mood improved. He will no doubt require this medication for some time yet, if not possibly forever.

One of our ongoing issues is the one of his smoking in the bedroom/ensuite. He continues to ignore my wishes in spite of our conversations about it. He said he knows I don't want him smoking there and he said he remembers when he does smoke upstairs how I feel about it. When I said I felt he was disrespectful of my wishes, he stared at me and offered no response. There are many health reasons why he shouldn't smoke; I have ignored those. There are also reasons why he shouldn't smoke in the bedroom. He ignores those. The reasons he continues, however, are likely those suggested by the ICBC therapist: rigidity, impulsiveness, lack of judgment, poor memory and perseverance (a dog with a bone attitude); all symptoms of frontal lobe injury.

He had become more motivated as he became interested in building his workshop. He was beginning to get a few small jobs doing what he did before his accident. This greatly helped his spirits and he appears to be much happier when he is busier. He is aware that he won't be able to go back to doing what he did before but he can certainly handle the smaller jobs and he derives some satisfaction from this.

Larry still becomes affected by 'bumps in the road' so we are still in a process of steps forward and backward. He may always be affected by 'bumps'. But all in all, I believe he has done well considering his injuries. I also believe that having him do cognitive exercises at an early stage after his injuries increased his recovery at a quicker rate than may have happened had he received no cognitive therapy until a later date.

Since Larry's accident, and no doubt as a result of his brain injury, he rarely says 'thank you' for anything and never says 'I'm sorry'. When asked if he thinks an 'I'm sorry' might be appropriate, he cannot see where he has done or said anything wrong. I hope over time his brain will repair itself to the extent he will realize when he has been in error. If not, this will no doubt be one of the deficits I will have to learn to accept.

I'm sure there will be many things we will have to learn to deal with; his inability to cope when things don't go well, resulting in his frustration, anger and irritability; his tendency to be self-centered; rigidity in his thinking; being unmotivated and his memory difficulties. These deficits are all symptoms of frontal lobe injury.

When Larry mentioned that he knew there was something different in his head than before, I mentioned his new awareness to his therapist. She said this was a great step forward. She said she had been at a stale-mate because he insisted that everything was fine. With this attitude, she said it would be very difficult to work on ways to adapt to the deficits. (He continued to deny his deficits to her). She said that denial is quite often a grieving process and some people will never be able to admit to having a brain injury or any deficits. She said perhaps when he learns new skills to adapt to the deficits things may become more similar to what they were.

She said both of us have been going through a grieving process. She said mine is the loss of what we once had. Admittedly, that had been bothering me considerably because I was slowly being forced to admit to myself that things may never be the same. I had in the beginning optimistically thought they might be if I worked hard enough with him. It has helped and I'm sure things are better than they would have been had I not.

Although he may never be the person he was before his accident, who he has become is better than the alternative might have been. There may still be times when I will have to remember not to take things personally when Larry is going through a frustrated period; and there may also be times ahead where it will be two steps forward and one step back. I do feel, however, that the steps backwards may be becoming fewer in frequency. I am beginning to see a glimmer of the 'old Larry' and over time hopefully he will learn to cope with the many 'bumps' there are in every road.

QUESTIONS I ASKED LARRY:

Q - Do you have any concerns about me writing this book about you?

A - No. It might help someone else.

Q - Do you have any memory of the accident?

A - No. I don't remember anything of that day at all – not getting up or making phone calls or leaving the house.

Q - How far back can you remember?

A - I don't remember anything until they moved me in with the three guys (almost six weeks after the accident) but even my whole hospital stay is vague.

Q - Do you have any memory of when you were so confused?

A - No. I don't remember being confused or saying strange things.

Q - Looking back, do you recall when you couldn't remember people when they came to visit you?

A - I don't remember any visitors during that time. And I don't remember actually getting moved in with the guys either. I think I may have still been confused.

A Roller Coaster Ride With Brain Injury (For Loved Ones)

Q - Do you remember being moved to Queen's Park Care Centre?

A - I don't remember the actual move although I do remember being in an ambulance and it hit the curb. I remember I was in with three older women before I was moved into a room of my own.

Q - Do you recall any of your difficult behavior either when you were at Royal Columbian Hospital or at Queen's Park Care Center?

A - Not specifically. I do remember when Meg was there (at Queen's Park) and you both left. I thought I may have been a little out of line but I didn't think I was too bad.

Q - Do you recall feeling frustrated and angry at Royal Columbian Hospital and Queen's Park Care Centre? Did some people or things make you more angry and frustrated than others did?

A - I was frustrated and angry all the time. I wasn't very happy there. The doctor made me angry and I thought I should have been doing therapy but nothing was happening. I just sat in bed all day.

Q - It appeared as if you were taking your anger and frustration out of me.

A - I don't know why I seemed to take my anger and frustration out on you – in the mornings I always looked forward to seeing you.

A Roller Coaster Ride With Brain Injury (For Loved Ones)

Q - Why did you refuse to stay off your feet, even knowing that you could cause more damage which may have meant you'd have to stay longer in the hospital?

A - I don't recall getting up at Royal Columbian Hospital. I do remember at Queen's Park but only when I had to go to the bathroom. I tried to avoid putting weight on my left leg when I used the walker. I tried to put the bulk of my weight on my right leg.

Q - Were you aware that you were potentially harming yourself?

A - I don't remember much from being at Royal Columbian Hospital so I have no idea why I did anything.

Q - When you were at Queen's Park Care Centre, were you aware you were depressed or were you capable of that much awareness?

A - I don't know if I was depressed or just plain angry and frustrated.

Q - Did you feel that coming home was a bit of a let-down?

A - I don't know if let-down is the proper word. Because I had been out of the loop for so long, I felt a little uncomfortable. I felt more like a guest than that I was at home. I wasn't comfortable in conversation either. It took a while to get over that feeling. I still feel

A Roller Coaster Ride With Brain Injury (For Loved Ones)

frustrated that I can't do what I want to do.

Q - You had some very difficult days after you came home – mood-wise – do you have any idea why you were feeling this way?

A - I remember that I did but I don't know why. You got the brunt of it because you were the one who was around.

Q - When you were in Queen's Park Care Centre, did you feel that you were not thinking and feeling as you should have been – in other words – did you feel in any way that you had a brain injury?

A - I knew I wasn't feeling myself but I didn't connect it to having a brain injury.

Q - How do you feel in this respect now? Can you feel there has been an improvement in your thinking and feelings?

A - It feels like there has been an improvement. I don't know whether it's an improvement in my brain injury or whether it's because I feel more comfortable. I feel like I live here and am not just a guest.

Q - From a mental viewpoint, not physical, do you feel there is a difference in your thinking and how you feel about things since your accident?

A - I still get frustrated and I don't know how

much I want to admit it has to do with a brain injury.

Q - Do you think you have changed somewhat since the accident, i.e.: do you think your tolerance level is the same? Are you more easily angered or frustrated than before?

A - I don't know if my tolerance level is the same. I do feel that I am more easily annoyed with the kids than I was previously.

Q - Have you noticed any changes that you are aware of since the accident?

A - No.

Q - Do you still enjoy socializing in the same way you did before your accident?

A - Yes, except I get uncomfortable because of my legs if I sit for a period of time.

Q - I have noticed that you are often quieter and don't often initiate conversations. Are you aware of this yourself?

A - It's the same thing as when I first came home – I felt as if I was out of the loop and

didn't know what was going on. I feel now that I know what is going on. (We are now getting the Province on a daily basis and I think this has contributed a lot to Larry's effort to participate more in conversations).

A Roller Coaster Ride With Brain Injury (For Loved Ones)

Larry initially had no inclination to read my story but later he listened while I read it to him. I told him I was going to tell it like it was and wasn't pulling any punches. He had no problem with that he said, if it helps someone else.

EXERCISES SIMILAR TO THOSE LARRY DID A FEW WEEKS AFTER HIS INJURY

Some of the exercises were an Orientation Aid to help provide orienting information about his present situation: where they are and why, dates and times.

Another part of the exercises were to be used as a Memory Aid to provide a tool to help cue new memories he may have recently stored but was having difficulty remembering. It was also used to help retrieve personal information from the past to 'fill in gaps' in his memory and to reinforce the correct information.

A third part of the exercises were used as a Therapy Aid which helped to work on other types of skills such as: thinking skills such as organization and summarizing, writing, reading for meaning and making sentences.

Several times a day I asked him very basic questions such as: What is the month, day and date and year? Where are you? Why are you here? Do you remember what you had for breakfast? How much of it did you eat? Do you remember what you had for lunch? Do you remember what you had for dinner? Do you remember who came in to visit you today?

A Roller Coaster Ride With Brain Injury (For Loved Ones)

Larry had a lot of trouble initially with these questions. For several weeks he thought it was 1996 instead of 2006 and the month, day and date were even more difficult for him to remember. For six or seven weeks he could not remember what he had eaten for any of his meals or who had visited him even when the visitor had left only a short time previously.

Other questions dealt with basic personal information and were asked until he remembered or knew the answers. Some of the questions were: When is your birthday? (he seemed to remember this) How old are you now? (he had difficulty with this one because he thought it was 1996) Where were you born? What is your address? (because of his move two months before his accident, he always gave his previous address) What is your phone number? (this was the same because of the move) How many children do you have? What are your children's names? What are your parents' names? Where do you work? Where have you traveled? How many siblings do you have? What are their names? Do you have any pets? What is your favorite T.V. show? What is your favorite sport? What is your favorite food? Why are you here? (he was unable to answer this for some time) Where are you? (he never really did know where he was either while he was in Royal Columbian or Queens Park Care Center)

Also, because he thought it was 1996, where he worked was another difficult question to answer correctly. Because he thought it was 1996 I did not ask him what his wife's name was. Although he

A Roller Coaster Ride With Brain Injury (For Loved Ones)

always knew my name, I have no idea if he was aware of where I fit into his life. He always seemed to expect me to be there so he somehow had rationalized my presence in his mind. This was very puzzling to me.

Other basic questions were:

Today is?... ... ...

Yesterday was?... ... ...

The day before yesterday was?... ... ...

Tomorrow will be?... ... ...

The day after tomorrow will be?... ... ...

The day before Monday is?... ... ...

How many days are in a year?... ... ...

How many months in a year?... ... ...

How many years in a century?... ... ...

Which months have 30 days?... ... ...

How many days are in the current month? ... ...

How often do we have a leap year?... ... ...

What is the third month of the year?... ... .

A Roller Coaster Ride With Brain Injury (For Loved Ones)

What is the eighth month of the year?... ... ...

What month is before January?... ... ...

What month was it five months ago?... ... ...

June falls in what season?... ... ...

Which season is the warmest?... ... ...

What holiday occurs in the Fall?... ... ...

What is your favorite time of the year and why?... ... ...

....

....

EXERCISES

No. 1 – Please answer the following questions:

	1	2	3	4
A	Pretty	Here	Dirty	Play
B	Child	Ugly	Story	Problem

What word is in space A4?... ... ...

Which word is to the right of Story?... ... ...

Which word is to the left of Ugly?... ... ...

A Roller Coaster Ride With Brain Injury (For Loved Ones)

What is the third word in Line B?... ... ...

How many words are in Line A following the word Here?... ... ...

Which word is next to Pretty?... ... ...

Which words are associated with toys?... ... ...
... ...

What word is the opposite of Ugly?... ... ...

Which words start with P?... ... ...
....

Which word is the opposite of Clean?... ... ...

What is the second word in Line A?... ... ...

What word is the opposite of Work?... ... ...

What word rhymes with Fear?... ... ...

How many words have the letter 'r' in them?
... ...

How many words are there in row A and B?
... ...

No. 2 – Please write the following series of words in their proper order.

Example:

loves   misery   company

A Roller Coaster Ride With Brain Injury (For Loved Ones)

Misery loves company

1. well   ends   all's   that

....

2. is   happiness   puppy   a   warm

....

3. makes   perfect   practice

....

4. not   want   waste   not

....

5. spoken   were   never   words   truer

....

6. love   do   I   how   thee

....

7. as   does   is   pretty   pretty

....

A Roller Coaster Ride With Brain Injury (For Loved Ones)

8. another   to   thing   one   leads

....

9. stitch   time   nine   in   saves   a

....

10. rod   child   spoil   the   spare   the

....

No. 3 – Use the information in the table below to answer the questions that follow:

Name	Age	Sex	Address
Sandra Shoemaker	12	F	2121 Elliot St.
Jennifer Solomon	13	F	6570 Hornet Dr.
Richard Jacobsen	10	M	7412 Holbrook St.
Sally Johnson	10	F	530 Holbrook St.

Name	Age	Sex	Address
Jacob Richardson	12	M	1541 Elliot Drive

Which boys live on Holbrook Street?... ... ...

... ...

How many girls are listed?... ... ...

A Roller Coaster Ride With Brain Injury (For Loved Ones)

How many boys are listed?... ... ...

List the children who are over 9 years of age and live on Holbrook Street? ... ...

....

    List the girls whose last names begin with "S".

....

....

Write the last names of each child in alphabetical order:..

....

....

....

Name	Age	Sex	Address
Donald McMillan	10	M	1212 Elmway Dr.
Robert McDonald	12	M	2450 Elmway Dr.
Patricia O'Malley	13	F	4517 Forest Dr.
Mary Murdoch	11	F	3450 Pine Cresc.
Peter Robertson	12	M	417 Forest Cresc.

List the girls whose last names begin with "M"

....

A Roller Coaster Ride With Brain Injury (For Loved Ones)

List all the boys who live on a 'Drive'..
....

Write the boys' first names in alphabetical order.

....
....

Which girls are over 10 and live on Forest Drive?... ... ...

5. How many boys' first name begins with an 'R'?... ... ...

PROBLEM SOLVING QUESTIONS

No. 1 – Read the list below and answer the following questions:

Light a match	Watch T.V.
Bake cookies	Tie a knot
Use scissors	Hammer nails
Play cards	File finger nails
Use an electric knife	Start a fire
Throw a baseball	Chew gum
Climb a ladder	Wrap a present

A Roller Coaster Ride With Brain Injury (For Loved Ones)

Write a letter	Telephone a friend
Walk down stairs	Peel a banana
Drive a car	Ride in a bus
Fix an engine	Sing a song
Fry chicken	Ride a bike
Go to a move	Walk uphill

Looking at the above list, what would be difficult to do but not dangerous if your arm was broken?... ... ...

... ...

....

....

....

....

Looking at the above list, write down the things that would be dangerous to do if your arm was broken..

....

....

A Roller Coaster Ride With Brain Injury (For Loved Ones)

No. 2 – Think about the following questions and answer to the best of your ability.

You are in the market for a new car. You find a car you may be interested in buying. What questions would you ask the car dealer about the car?

....

....

....

....

You are looking for an apartment to rent. List what you need to know about the apartment and the location before making a decision to rent it.

....

....

....

....

You visit your doctor because you've been experiencing persistent headaches.

What would be important things to tell or ask your doctor?

....

A Roller Coaster Ride With Brain Injury (For Loved Ones)

....

....

....

You plan to buy a house and think you have found one you like. What are important things to know before making your final decision?

....

....

....

....

You are at an interview for a position in your field. What kind of questions would you ask your future employer?

....

....

....

No. 3 – Read the story below aloud. Then cover the story and answer the following questions. Try to remember the main facts in the story as you read it.

A Roller Coaster Ride With Brain Injury (For Loved Ones)

The small town of Salmon Arm in the Interior of British Columbia is home to the many houseboats that travel the Shuswap Lake from late Spring until mid-Fall. Many tourists travel by houseboat along the lake shore and beyond, often in large groups or in their own small party. The experience is enjoyable to most unless you happen to be one of the unlucky ones to be caught in one of the summer storms that sometimes spring out of nowhere. At that time boats can run aground or capsize if they are out on the lake. There are rules that must be followed for everyone's safety. Some of those rules are: If a wind comes up, you are to return to shore and anchor and tie your boat; everyone must wear life jackets; staying in a group offers protection and look out for your fellow boater.

What town is this story about? … … … … … ……

What is the name of the lake?
....

When do the tourists come to this town?
....

What is a popular attraction for the tourists to this small town?

....

....

What can sometimes suddenly happen on the lake?
....

A Roller Coaster Ride With Brain Injury (For Loved Ones)

....

At that time what must each boater be aware of?

....

What are some of the rules?
....

....

....

No. 4 – Read the story below aloud. Then cover it and try to answer the questions that follow. Try to remember as many of the facts in the story as possible.

As a photographer, Adam traveled throughout British Columbia to take pictures of the mountains, lakes, rivers and the many Gulf Islands. Many of the places he traveled were serene where nature was at its best. These were the areas he enjoyed the most particularly when the ocean was not far away. He liked to stay away from the cities with their pollution and concrete. Blue skies and ocean waves were his loves.

What did Adam do for a living?
....
Where did he travel?
....

A Roller Coaster Ride With Brain Injury (For Loved Ones)

What did he love the most?

....

What didn't he like?

....

What did he take pictures of?

....

No. 5 – Have someone read each memory exercise to you having you answer each question.

When Maureen got home from work, she laid her purse, keys and coat on the chair in the corner of the family room. That evening she hung up her coat and put her purse in the bedroom.

The next morning she was unable to find her keys. Where were they?

....

Stephen went to the store to buy five grocery items. He needed milk, coffee, hot chocolate, marshmallows and jam. When he got home he discovered that he had only bought four of the items.

He bought the milk, coffee, hot chocolate and jam. What had he forgotten?

....

Several men were planning a fishing trip. Their names were David, Cameron and Mike. David was

A Roller Coaster Ride With Brain Injury (For Loved Ones)

driving with the fishing gear. First he picked up Mike who had the camping equipment.

Whom did he pick up next?... ... ...

A car salesman was discussing the purchase of a used Monte Carlo with a customer. There were three available. A 1979 model was $7,400.00, a 1981 model was $5,400.00 and a 1983 model was $8,400.00.

How much did the 1981 model cost?... ... ...

You are going to buy supplies to make a bookcase but first you have to take the measurements, see how much wood you already have and check your nail supply.

What do you have to do before you buy your supplies?... ... ...

....

....

When you go on vacation, you have to cancel your mail, water your plants and take out the garbage.

What do you have to do before you go on vacation?... ... ...

....

As a witness to an accident, the policeman asked if you remembered the direction the second

A Roller Coaster Ride With Brain Injury (For Loved Ones)

car was going, the condition of the road and the time of day so you can testify in court.

What are you supposed to remember?... ... ...

... ...

....

Your dental hygienist told you to brush your teeth two times daily, floss once daily and not to chew ice.

What did she tell you?... ... ...

... ...

....

Your wife's friend calls to say that the golf game planned for Saturday is still on but the time has been changed from 1:30 p.m. to 12:30 p.m. and she will meet your wife in the parking lot.

What did your wife's friend say?... ... ...

....
....

....

You call the bank to ask what their hours are on Friday, if they're open on Saturday and what is the cost of a safe-deposit box.

A Roller Coaster Ride With Brain Injury (For Loved Ones)

What do you want to ask?... ... ...

....

....

No. 6 – Explain what you would do in each of the following situations:

Your dog bit a neighbor's child

....

....

....

You overslept and missed an important appointment..

....

....

You mistakenly made plans with two different people for the same evening. What would you do?

....

....

....

You locked your keys in your car?
....

A Roller Coaster Ride With Brain Injury (For Loved Ones)

....

You suspected that your child took his grandmother's blood pressure medication?

....

....

Your spouse was an hour later getting home from work than she said she would be?..

....

....

A neighbor calls angrily to tell you that your child has hit her child?

....

....

....

Your landlord gives you notice to move. It is insufficient notice.

....

....

You begin to receive anonymous phone calls.

A Roller Coaster Ride With Brain Injury (For Loved Ones)

....

....

No. 7 – Study the following 12 items for several minutes. Then cover them and write down as many as you can remember in the spaces provided.

Monday	Thursday
Dodge	Nissan
Tuesday	Chrysler
two	Saturday
Honda	six
five	three

All of the above items belong in three categories. Write the three categories in the space below:

....

....

....

....

The three categories:..................................

....

A Roller Coaster Ride With Brain Injury (For Loved Ones)

DIRECTIONS: Write the words that match the numbers.

Example: lamb   Mary   a   little   had
             5   1   3   4   2

          Mary had a little lamb.
           1   2   3   4   5

1.   well   ends   all's   that
       2 & 5   4   1   3

_____

2.
  .   want   waste   not
        1   3   2 & 4

_____

DIRECTIONS: Answer the following questions as completely as possible.

Imagine you are sitting beside a stranger. You would like to get to know him. What questions would you ask?

_____

_____

_____

A Roller Coaster Ride With Brain Injury (For Loved Ones)

You are in the market for a new car. You find one you may be interested in. What questions would you ask the car dealer?

You are looking for an apartment to rent. List what you need to consider before renting one?

A Roller Coaster Ride With Brain Injury (For Loved Ones)

			May			
S	M	T	W	T	F	S
	1	2	3	4	5	6
7	8	9	10	11	12	13
14	15	16	17	18	19	20
21	22	23	24	25	26	27
28	29	30	31			

Directions: Fill the Dates to Remember on the calendar with the information listed below:

Doctor's appointment – 1:30 p.m. – May 23rd
Sister's birthday dinner – 5:00 p.m. – May 14th
Job interview – 10:00 a.m. – May 25th
Mortgage payment due – May 1st
Hair appointment – 9:00 a.m. - May 30th
Son's soccer game – 6:00 p.m. – May 22nd
Wife's/Husbands birthday – May 17th
Lunch with friend – 12:30 p.m. – May 5th

A Roller Coaster Ride With Brain Injury (For Loved Ones)

EXERCISE DIRECTIONS: Study a picture for 50 seconds. Then cover the picture and ask the following questions:

1. What was going on in the picture?
2. What type of buildings, if any, did you notice?
3. Approximately how many people were in the picture?
4. What were they doing?
5. Were there any animals in the picture?
6. How would you describe the area (suburban, rural, etc.)?
7. If there were people – how many were men?
8. Women?
9. Children?
10. If there were buildings, were they small, medium or large?
11. How many trees were in the yard?
12. Were there any children playing outside?
13. Were there any vehicles in the picture?

As the memory improves, increase the complexity of the questions asked about the pictures used.

MEMORY EXERCISE: Have someone read each exercise and write down the answer. As memory improves allow more time before answering.

1. Before you leave home, you must remember to bring the cat in, turn off the stove, turn off the lights and lock the door.

....

....

A Roller Coaster Ride With Brain Injury (For Loved Ones)

2. When you go to the store you must pick up bread, pickles, cereal and toilet paper.

   ....

   ....

3. You want to remember to tell your friend that Jake called, you'll meet at the movies at 3:00 p.m. and you have to do an errand first.

   ....

   ....

4. The doctor told you to do exercises every day, to take a daily multivitamin and to eat lots of fruit and vegetables.

   ....

   ....

ISBN 1425169643